The Ties that Bind: Men's and Women's Social Networks

The *Marriage & Family Review* series:

- *Family Medicine: A New Approach to Health Care*, edited by Betty E. Cogswell and Marvin B. Sussman

- *Cults and the Family*, edited by Florence Kaslow and Marvin B. Sussman

- *Intermarriage in the United States*, edited by Gary A. Cretser and Joseph J. Leon

- *Alternatives to Traditional Family Living*, edited by Harriet Gross and Marvin B. Sussman

- *Family Systems and Inheritance Patterns*, edited by Judith N. Cates and Marvin B. Sussman

- *The Ties that Bind: Men's and Women's Social Networks*, edited by Laura Lein and Marvin B. Sussman

The Ties that Bind: Men's and Women's Social Networks

Laura Lein and Marvin B. Sussman
Editors

Marriage & Family Review
Volume 5, Number 4

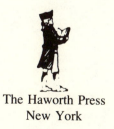

The Haworth Press
New York

The Haworth Press, Inc., 28 East 22 Street, New York, NY 10010

Library of Congress Cataloging in Publication Data
Main entry under title:

The Ties that bind.

(Marriage & family review ; v. 5, no. 4)
Includes bibliographical references.
1. Social structure—Addresses, essays, lectures. 2. Social interaction—Addresses, essays, lectures. 3. Parents—Addresses, essays, lectures. 4. Aged—Addresses, essays, lectures. 5. Poor—Addresses, essays, lectures. I. Lein, Laura. II. Sussman, Marvin B. III. Series.
HM131.T52   1983   305   82-23230
ISBN 0-86656-161-7

The Ties that Bind:
Men's and Women's Social Networks

Marriage & Family Review
Volume 5, Number 4

CONTENTS

Editor's Note

Social networks are coming into prominence as viable sources of help, support, affection, warmth, love, and solidarity. These have existed and functioned for eons of time handling the problems, deviancies, torts, anxieties, and socialization of their members. The new importance of these networks as functional service systems is a result of decreasing support for institutional professionalized human services—a turn to self-help and increased involvement in caring and other helping activities by members of such primary groups as families.

It is easy to conceptualize the family as the unit of linkage and analysis in social network research. It is extremely difficult to characterize and measure family networking. Network studies focus on individual member's connections, and some of these serve the person or, in some instances, purport to represent the family. The individual's networking at times presumes an other-than-self interest, but differentiating the objectives and functions of networks for the individual or family's benefit is a difficult, if not an impossible, task.

One approach used extensively is the analysis of the social networks of members within the family, e.g., the mother-child, grandparent-grandchild, nephew-aunt relationships. These intrafamily connections are examined in relation to their impact on activities, functions, quality of life, and other behavioral outcomes. Another approach is to view individual family members' network activities with individuals and representatives of non-family groups and bureaucracies in relation to personal agendas or family interests. How much is personal or family depends on the roles assumed by family members and expectations of performance of these roles. The individual who has achieved or been ascribed the role of family representative to the school bureaucracy will network with representatives of other family members to develop an optimal connectedness with the educational institution which benefits the child and the family. Networking for support and help when there is a chronic illness of a family member may result in relief for the principal caretaker with obvious consequences for other family members. The caretaker may be able to return to normal roles thus easing the workload of other family members.

The activities of networks of men and women are neither solely for personal gain and isolated from family, except in the case of the single-person household, nor are they completely performed for the family. These networks represent in varying proportions the individual and family interests and concerns. The situation, purpose, rationale, motivation, and interest of the network participant determine who are the potential beneficiaries of network activities and the proportional distribution of benefits for the individual or the group. The reader should consider these notions when reading articles on networks active in different life sectors.

Marvin B. Sussman

The Ties That Bind:
An Introduction

Laura Lein

Social networks, "a specified set of links among social actors" (Fischer et al., 1977, p. 33), have become a significant focus of research in the last two decades. Social networks represent a "web of association" for individuals in the larger society. They have been described as follows:

> Individuals are linked to their society primarily through relations with other individuals: with kin, friends, co-workers, fellow club members, and so on. We are each the center of a web of social bonds that radiates outward to the people whom we know intimately, those whom we know well, those whom we know casually, and to the wider society beyond. These are our personal social networks. Society affects us largely through tugs on the strands of our networks—shaping our attitudes, providing opportunities, making demands on us and so forth. And it is by tugging at those same strands that we make our individual impacts on society—influencing other people's opinions, obtaining favors from "insiders," forming action groups. (Fischer, p. vii)

The study of social networks provides not only a model of society useful to social scientists, but represents an important part of everyone's daily lives. The social network is the arena in which social life occurs. Attitudes and beliefs are formed and shaped by interaction with network members. Goods and services for meeting day-to-day and emergency needs are often obtained in the same way. Not only do networks allow individuals to provide each other

Laura Lein is Director of the Wellesley College Center for Research on Women. Work on this volume was partially supported by NIMH Grant No. 29469.

with pragmatic and logistical help, but they provide emotional and psychological support.

Moreover, social networks are the source of demands and constraints on individuals, as well as supports and opportunities. Network members challenge beliefs as well as support them, make demands for services as well as provide them, and close off opportunities as well as open them. Through gossip, the threat of ostracism, and the withdrawal of support, social networks can punish unconventional behavior. Because so many aspects of individual life are affected by social networks, social scientists continue to examine them as a way of understanding how "social forces" affect individual and family activities and how individuals and families, in turn, make their mark on the neighborhood, community, and larger society.

As many have pointed out, sociology has become a discipline engaged primarily in the study of institutions (e.g., Kanter, 1977). There is a sociology of work, of family, of community, of organizations, and so on. While this may be a convenient way to divide the social universe for the sake of studying it, it does not reflect the reality of the lives of individuals who must juggle multiple and overlapping responsibilities and affiliations. Analysis of social networks provides a conceptualization of social life that illuminates the ties among the different spheres of an individual's social world.

It is a truism that women's life experiences, needs for social supports, and social worlds differ appreciably from those of men. There are important human conditions and events that are particular to women: pregnancy, childbirth, greater vulnerability to sexual abuse. In addition, men and women have traditionally assumed different roles and functions in the family, the labor force, and the wider community. Men's and women's roles affect the demands each make on social networks, their opportunities to build support networks, and the services and supports they can offer to network members in exchange.

Men's and women's traditional roles include a sex-based division of labor in the participation and support of social networks. Women have largely born responsibility for maintaining family ties to church and kin groups, the neighborhood and community organizations (especially those related to children's activities and schooling). Men have been more likely to use paid work and community-based peer groups as the focus of their friendships and socializing.

However, men's and women's roles are shifting with changes in the demography of family life. More women, in particular more women with young children, hold paid jobs outside the home. More couples postpone the onset of parenthood and limit family size. More people survive to very old age, and the gap in life expectancy between women and men is widening. Such changes raise new questions about how the support systems of men and women respond to changes in responsibility and how these changing demands on men and women, in turn, reshape the organization and functioning of their social networks. The differences in men's and women's, boys' and girls' social networks affect most other arenas of their lives.

When men's and women's roles are undergoing considerable change and examination, it is important to understand the ways in which individuals, both men and women, negotiate their family involvements and their work and community commitments. Family, work, community, church, and other institutions include individual members who are tied to each other both by the fact of their formal membership in the same institution and by their place in each other's social networks. Men's and women's different affiliations, as well as the differences in their activities and responsibilities, lead to differences in their social networks. Network analysis has enabled scholars to come to a better understanding of the impact of social networks on men's and women's lives.

In this volume each author explores the social networks of men and women under different life circumstances, facing different demands, and requiring different resources. Lydia O'Donnell discusses the social networks of men and women during the parenting years. She reviews the literature on parents' needs for social supports, on the kinds of supports they customarily receive through social networks, on the contributions made by parents to social networks, and on the role of children in the social networks of their parents.

Ann Stueve writes of the position of the elderly in each other's social networks and in the social networks of younger individuals. She shows how the customary focus on the elderly as the beneficiaries of services must be modified by their significance as contributors through social networks.

Michelene Malson explores the literature on the social networks of Black families. She discusses the theories of Black families' support networks and Black families' economic maintenance. She suggests the variations among Black families.

Deborah Belle examines the literature on the social networks of poor families. She discusses the relationship between social networks and such factors as stress, psychological well-being, and family economic maintenance.

Several qualities of social networks make their study particularly intriguing. First, unlike groups with well-defined boundaries, networks are much more amorphous, radiating outward with fluid boundaries. Second, different parts of a person's network can exist somewhat separately from one another. An individual, for example, may have one group of friends at work, another through her church, and another through the PTA and her children's schoolmates. Each of these parts of her network may or may not overlap. Finally, networks are never static. New members are added and old members drop out, some to return again later. Many of these changes occur with life transitions such as marriage or career changes; others are more gradual.

There are two common approaches to describing and characterizing social networks. First, one can focus on network composition, that is, the characteristics of network members. Research here tends to raise the question, "Who is in one's network? How does network composition vary across social groups? How does it vary across other individual social and demographic parameters?" Second, researchers focus on network processes, the functioning and different attributes of dyadic links between network members.

In 1957, Bott published a seminal work, the book *Family and Social Network*. Through a series of detailed interviews with twenty English families, all with at least one child under ten years at home, she explored the relationship between that most intimate part of most individuals' social network, the family, and the composition of the family's kinship and friendship networks. More specifically, she suggested that families where men's and women's roles and activities are relatively sex-segregated possess what she termed close-knit networks. Families with looser networks possess a more companionate model of family life. Gary R. Lee (1979) has presented a more recent and equally exhaustive review on the "Effects of Social Networks on the Family." He begins with Bott and then explores the schools of research which have emerged from the themes she initiated.

Since Bott's earlier work, there has been immense development of the literature on men's and women's social networks. We have learned that men and women possess different kinds of social networks and feel different kinds of obligations to members of their social networks. Both of these facts have powerful implications for the lives of men and women in the family, in the workplace, and in the larger community. In addition, because men and women have different kinds of social networks, they are supported in different kinds of activities and.roles.

This can become a difficulty for both men and women as their traditionally defined responsibilities in the home and in the workplace change. Men need new kinds of support to enable them to participate more fully in family life. Similarly, women need new kinds of social networks to enable them to participate fully in the paid labor force. This volume explores aspects of men's and women's social networks: the important functions of networks, and the ways social networks shape adult lives at different points in the life cycle and for men and women in different kinds of families.

In this volume, the reviews explore the implications of social networks for men and women in several significant social contexts. However, each review is concerned with illustrating the links between network structure and network functioning, and the changes in networks as individuals change circumstances.

The Social Worlds of Parents

Lydia O'Donnell

Not only do parents play a major role in structuring their children's social interactions and relationships with the world outside the home, but children, in turn, influence the social worlds of parents, by shaping both their intimate and informal involvements with family, friends, and neighbors, and their more formal and less personal engagements within the wider community. As a small but growing number of researchers is beginning to recognize, this influence begins before the birth of a first child and continues, to greater or lesser degrees, throughout the subsequent stages of parenting.

The difficulties—and joys—of raising children pull parents in directions different from those of non-parents. Parents tend to seek out the support and companionship of other adults who are at similar points in the child-rearing cycle and who are confronted with similar situations and stresses. Parents of special-needs children and single parents who are raising children alone also seem to gravitate toward each other, molding their social networks to fit their particular needs for companionship and support. The role of children in shaping the social worlds of their parents, moreover, is not limited to the active and early stages of child-rearing. Having children who are grown also makes a difference for men and women in old age. Elderly parents are more likely to maintain a greater number of contacts with both the middle and younger (grandchild) generations than non-parents; they are also less likely to be placed in institutions for the old. (See Stueve, in this issue.)

Despite the widespread acknowledgement and the obvious statement that children radically transform their parents' lives, there have been few systematic efforts to document either the variety of ways in which children structure the informal relations and formal

---

Lydia O'Donnell is a graduate student at the Graduate School of Education, Harvard University.

ties of their parents or the ways in which these relations and ties evolve as children grow older. This is hardly surprising, given the fact that attention has only recently turned to issues of adult development and socialization. As sociologists and psychologists have pointed out, we know far more about how parents affect the lives of children than how children affect the lives of their parents (e.g., Bell, 1968; Bell and Harper, 1977; Rapoport et al., 1979).

To date, work conducted on the topic of child influences on adults has been primarily limited to one of two frameworks. The first is largely psychological in approach. For example, there has been a growing awareness that in order to understand the process of parent-infant bonding, we must not only study how mothers and fathers treat and influence their infants, but how infants shape the behavior of their parents (e.g., Lewis and Rosenblum, 1974), and how family members, taken together, operate as a "system of reciprocal and interacting influences that change over time" (Parke and Savin, 1980, p. 46). Unfortunately, most of the work relying on this model is still limited to an examination of personal relations within the mother-father-infant triad and during the earliest stages of child-rearing. The few studies which include older children focus on child effects on adult behaviors (such as verbal responses), but not on the construction of parents' social worlds (e.g., Osofosky and O'Connell, 1972; Yarrow et al., 1971). The second framework is more sociological and thus more directly concerned with how children affect the social worlds of their parents. However, it has thus far tended to focus on the constraints children impose on parents', and particularly mothers', lives (e.g., Bernard, 1974; Sokoloff, 1980). While this line of research has been instrumental in helping us understand the detrimental effects of child care responsibilities on women's labor force participation, status attainment, and the like, it often ignores the many ways children also enrich and augment their parents' lives and social interactions.

For example, Schraneveldt and Ihinger (1979) suggest that children open up the family system by rendering more permeable the boundaries both between subunits of the extended family and between families and the wider community. The social implications of these changes are discussed by Slater (1964), who argues that parenthood is one important mechanism for preventing couples from remaining in overly intense and exclusive dyadic bonds. It does so "by creating responsibilities and obligations which are partly societal in nature, and through which bonds between the dyad and the community are thereby generated" (p. 240). Indeed, evidence from survey studies suggests that parents in the active stages of child-rearing are more likely to be involved in their neighborhoods and communities than either childless individuals or parents whose children have come of age (Fischer et al., 1977).

While social scientists have always been interested in the nature and consequences of social relations, few studies have examined the social worlds of parents directly. This is in part due to the fact that it is only in recent years that the construct of a social network and its associated terminology have come into vogue. (For a discussion, see Lewis and Weinraub, 1976.) As a result, the literature pertaining to parenting and social networks is scattered across a variety of research areas, with a resulting inconsistency of perspective, terminology, methodology, and depth. In this review, I attempt to pull together and discuss what is known about how children, from birth through school-age, shape the social involvements of their parents. I draw upon a wide range of resources, including older studies of family and community life, research which attempts to chart and account for variations in the social-network configurations of different groups, personal accounts of the parenting experience, and a growing literature which focuses on how social supports and networks contribute to and help alleviate the demands and strains of parenthood.

Because this is a first effort to integrate a widely scattered literature, I have imposed a number of limitations on the topics and populations discussed. First is the decision to limit the review to the most active stages of parenting, that is, when children are school-age or younger. The question of how teenagers and even adult children influence their parents' social worlds is certainly intriguing, but, as yet, it is largely unaddressed. Literature on adolescence, for example, focuses less on the intersections of parents' and teenagers' social worlds than on issues of separation and the emergence of independent social lives. Second, the review primarily focuses on white nuclear families, a limitation which reflects the bias of much of the available research. While a number of the studies cited here include married and single parents and both black and white families, I have not made an attempt to review those separate (and, in themselves, extensive) literatures on parenting alone, remarriage and "reconstituted" families, unwed parents or the child-rearing supports of black and other minority parents. Although it would be most useful to pull what is relevant from these literatures into a discussion of the social worlds of parents and to contrast the experiences of different groups, such a presentation is beyond the scope of the present paper.

An additional restriction is the lack of a full discussion of how the social worlds of parents are affected by the presence of a child with a serious disability. As Featherstone (1980) points out, "A special loneliness is the most pervasive theme in the stories told by parents with disabled children" (p. 50). Such a child can create both psychological and physical barriers to parents' participation in the normal web of human interactions. What other parents come to count on as normal supports, such as the help and shared excitement of grandparents, may be unavailable to the parents of a disabled child. Even when help is available, it may be insufficient to remove a parent's sense of desolation and isolation (Friedland and Kort, 1981). What men and women count on as the normal constraints and limitations imposed by parenthood become magnified:

> Disability may isolate families in a variety of ways. Most concretely it often interferes with ordinary social activities. Young children always complicate their parent's efforts to get out of the house. . . . A disability adds to the difficulty of organizing expeditions and recreation. It also creates invisible social barriers. (Featherstone, 1980, p. 51)

These barriers can seriously hamper the efforts of parents of a special-needs child to live so-called "normal" social lives. Women whose children need constant special care and training question whether they can take away the time and energy to hold down an outside paid job; both fathers and mothers question whether they can go about their daily routines, and whether they can manage to arrange for leisure time, either as individuals or as couples.

In summary, the review does not discuss in detail how the social worlds of parents change when men and women are faced with the demands of raising a child with special needs, of raising children alone, or of raising children under any of a number of other particular circumstances. It is necessary, however, to remember that adults' worlds are shaped not by the presence of some hypothetically typical children, but by the compelling and often idiosyncratic needs of their real life sons and daughters and by the circumstances in which they must parent. This is only a first attempt to collect and organize what we know about how children modify and contribute to their parent's social worlds. Only by beginning to address this question directly will we further our understanding of the demands, satisfactions, stresses, and rewards of parenting in a wide variety of circumstances.

I. ENTRY INTO PARENTHOOD

It has been almost fifteen years since Rossi (1968) reminded social scientists that parenting affects not only children but the adults involved as well. In her widely cited article "The Transition to Parenthood," she called for a new research agenda which would focus on how entry into parenthood as a social role reshapes the life commitments and social involvements of adults, and, in particular, the social worlds of women. At this point, we have amassed a considerable amount of information on how having a baby constrains and pulls a mother away from her previous activities and involvements; we know less, however, about how the social worlds of mothers are rebuilt and restructured in order to accommodate the demands of child care. We know still less about how being a new parent affects a father's social ties—to his extended family, his workplace, or to the community, and we are only beginning to sort out how variations in social networks and access to social supports shape the quality and types of interactions among mothers, fathers, and their infants.

The most abrupt and well-studied shift in life commitments which corresponds with the birth of a first child is the withdrawal of mothers from participation in the workplace. Despite the fact that most mothers will return to employment at some later point in their parenting careers, the majority of women terminate their employment to become, at least for a while, full-time homemakers (Shapiro and Mott, 1979; U.S. Department of Labor, 1973, 1979). A number of researchers have written about the sense of isolation and loss women experience when they retire from the structured public world of the office or factory and begin to redefine their work in terms of the needs of a child and home (e.g., Bernard, 1974; LeMasters, 1957; Lopata, 1971; Oakley, 1981). There can be a stressful period of time in which new mothers (particularly those residing in non-ethnic communities apart from an active kin network) feel dislocated and cut off from peers—the renegotiation of old ties and the building of new ones can take time. There is some evidence, from the personal accounts of new mothers, that the friendship of another woman who has recently experienced motherhood herself lessens this sense of aloneness and supports a woman in her efforts to assume and identify with her new maternal role. Unfortunately, there is little research which discusses the resiliency which is characteristic of many new mothers, or women's ability to establish different but rewarding networks in their neighborhoods and communities. For example, some women sustain and build upon the contacts they made while attending childbirth education classes; some seek out other mothers in their neighborhoods who are taking care of young infants (Friedland and Kort, 1981). Still others find being a full-time housewife and mother too confining, and return to paid employment not only for financial reasons but for the social opportunities it offers as well (Friedland and Kort, 1981; Oakley, 1980).

New fathers also experience a shift in the nature of their workplace commitments, although the nature and extent of this shift is not as well documented. There is clearly a jump in the family's economic needs and an increased emphasis on the man's breadwinning role. A survey of 162 highly educated husbands residing in a university community showed that while only 25% of "families in general" felt that husbands should be entirely responsible for the family's economic support, this proportion increased to 55% when the family in question was specified as having a young child not yet in school (Pleck et al., 1978). In the study by Grossman et al. (1980) of the pregnancy and first year postpartum experiences of 84 couples, expectant fathers were asked whether their wives' pregnancies had caused any changes in themselves. One father replied, "I guess you realize you're no longer a child yourself. I feel that in subtle ways, in regard to my work. . . . I feel more responsible in my job, more concerned about making enough money from it. I guess I feel good about it" (p. 166). In contrast, even when new mothers are employed, their income is more likely to be viewed as supplementary rather than essential, and the importance of their employment is likely to be downplayed (Entwisle and Doering, 1980; LaRossa and LaRossa, 1981).

With the birth of a child, men enter into what has been termed the male "life-cycle squeeze"; they are faced with a growing number of pressures to increase their involvements in both family life and the workplace (Oppenheimer, 1974). Unfortunately, the workplace appears to offer relatively little support to its male employees either in easing the transition to parenthood or in helping a man assume an active role in parenting as children grow. Several researchers have suggested that personal support from co-workers as well as institutional support such as parenting leaves and flexible schedules could play an important role in helping men balance the new demands of work and family life (Fein, 1974; Parke, n.d.).

In addition to redefining men's and women's commitments to the workplace, the transition to parenthood calls for a reformulation of many old personal relationships. A substantial literature exists on how children affect the relation between husband and wife (e.g., Hobbs, 1968; LeMasters, 1957; Meyerowitz and Feldman, 1966; Parke and O'Leary, 1975). This work primarily examines two outcomes, marital satisfaction and the household division of labor. (While there is some debate about whether household members should be considered part of one's network, most studies of parenting look at fathers as a potential source of support for mothers, the primary child-rearers.)

Despite decades of research, there is disagreement as to the overall impact of parenthood on a couple's marriage. (For a brief annotated bibliography, see LaRossa and LaRossa, 1980; see also Lerner and Spanier, 1978.) A number of cross-sectional comparisons of parents and childless couples have indicated that children reduce marital satisfaction, especially among wives (Brown, 1974; Campbell et al., 1976; Glenn, 1975; Glenn and Weaver, 1978; Rollins and Feldman, 1970). Other studies also suggest that a majority of couples appear to experience at least a "slight" crisis after they become parents. Yet, in contrast, they indicate that only a minority of parents feel that their marriages have deteriorated or become less satisfying since the birth of their first child (Hobbs and Cole, 1976; Russell, 1974). Furthermore, research by Rausch (1974) and his associates raises the possibility that communication between husbands and wives may actually improve with parenthood, perhaps because, as recently pointed out by Gilstrap et al. (1981), the demands of raising a child give a couple something new to talk about. Indeed, a number of studies now demonstrate that problems with pregnancy, delivery, or early care of an infant may actually increase marital communication and husband's involvement in family life (Gilstrap et al., 1981; Peterson, 1980).

The Cowans (1981) point to the inadequacy of many cross-sectional studies in informing us about how children affect the marital relationship and stress the need for more studies which look at men and women both before and after the birth of a child. Unfortunately, the high costs of longitudinal work seriously limit the number of men and women who can be interviewed. In their own longitudinal study of 27 couples, they report that fathers who were more involved in tending to the needs of their babies reported greater marital satisfaction. Women reported greater satisfaction the more their husbands participated in domestic and family chores, and the more they agreed with the division of child care responsibilities in the family. The association among actual patterns or division of labor, couples' satisfaction with the division of labor (whatever its style), and their overall appraisal of the marital relation is an interesting one, since numerous studies indicate that having a first child pulls couples into less egalitarian and more sex-typed domestic and employment roles (Entwisle and Doering, 1980; Hoffman, 1978; Hoffman and Manis, 1978; LaRossa and LaRossa, 1981). This raises the interesting research question of whether marital satisfaction is contingent upon a particular division of labor or whether it is more dependent upon couples' satisfaction with whatever they are doing, regardless of this division.

Entwisle and Doering's (1980) interviews with 120 wives (and many of their husbands) illustrate how, in moving towards traditional roles, couples decrease the pressure which would be caused by maintaining egalitarian and non-sex-typed values by mutually devaluing the women's paid-work role. In the LaRossas' (1981) study of 20 upper-middle class couples, the wife's employment was found to be the most important factor (over age of the parents, number of years married, and number of children) influencing the relationship between parenthood and family interactions. Yet the fact of employment was not what appeared to matter; what counted were such personal considerations and attitudes such as whether the wife was at home or at work voluntarily, whether her husband was supportive and sympathetic of her work situation, and what kind of ambivalence the couple felt about their arrangement of work and family roles.

In addition to influencing the marriage of their parents, the arrival of children also calls for a redefinition of other family relationships. Many women report that they grew closer to their own mothers after becoming a mother themselves. Certainly, grandmothers in our society make an effort to be on hand following the birth of their daughters' first children, and both grandmothers and grandfathers initiate patterns of support—emotional, material, and social—which continue throughout the early child-rearing years (Hill, 1970; Sussman, 1965). Although there is still much to be learned about how the informal networks of new parents vary by such characteristics as social class and ethnicity, a number of British and American ethnographic studies have demonstrated that closer ties usually exist between the grandparent and parent generations among working-class families; working-class daughters and their mothers appear to form a particularly close bond (e.g., Bott, 1957; Gans, 1967; Fried, 1973; Rubin, 1976; Young and Willmott, 1957). Oakley (1981), in her study titled *Becoming a Mother*, illustrates how much information about pregnancy, childbirth, and infant care is transmitted from working-class mothers to their adult daughters. Middle-class women may rely more heavily on written materials and self-help parenting guides.

Not all grandparents are perceived as welcome sources of help and support, at least at this earliest stage of parenting. At times they are depicted as drawing energy away from the mother-father-baby triad at a critical stage in nuclear-family formation and role development. In addition, their values and infant-care strategies may conflict with those of the new parents. Although this issue is rarely discussed in the academic literature, a number of popular parenting guides (usually aimed at middle-class audiences) advise couples to delay and limit grandparents' visits with the new family until the new parent-baby bonds are secure and both fathers and mothers are comfortable with their parenting roles (e.g., Gold and Gold, 1977; Hall, 1972). What these guides remind us of, in essence, is the time and energy entailed in maintaining social relations, even with those most intimate and known. What most research on early parenting points out (and what anyone who has lived through the experience knows) is how little of these commodities parents have left over after meeting the needs of their demanding new family member. Men interviewed in Dyer's (1963) study of middle-class couples with children aged two and younger, for example, mentioned the strain entailed in working out new arrangements with grandparents and other relatives as one of the major difficulties of becoming a father.

An additional change in the network involvements of new parents is their exposure to a new arena of professionals and self-help groups. This involvement begins prior to childbirth when contacts with obstetricians, childbirth educators, and pediatricians are initiated. Although childbirth education courses began as a largely middle-class phenomenon, use and acceptance of courses as support for the pregnancy and childbirthing experience have spread to working-class and low-income populations as well (see, for example, Entwisle's (1979) difficulty in finding non-course attenders). There is a growing amount of evidence which suggests that courses function as supports in two ways. First, the training received appears to facilitate the actual delivery, to involve fathers in the birthing process, to influence favorably both parents' perceptions of the birthing experience, and to facilitate parent-infant interactions following the birth (e.g., Entwisle and Doering, 1980; Peterson and Mehl, 1977). Second, the courses provide expectant parents with introductions to other couples in a similar life stage and serve as a first encounter with a parenting-support group (Cowan et al., 1978).

A final body of research focuses on the complex interactions among the social worlds of mothers and fathers, infant development, and parental stress. A product of the recent interest in ecological models for studying family life, this is the most rapidly expanding area of work relating to parenting and social networks. For example, Belsky and his colleagues have noted that three negative aspects of parents' social worlds—a sense of isolation, socially impoverished neighborhoods, and unemployment—correlate with occurrences of maladaptive child rearing such as child abuse. In their preliminary analyses, his research group has found unexpectedly few relationships between social-network measures and assessments of mother-infant interactions, but some differences for interactions between infants and first-time fathers. They suggest that peer support and contact with friends, neighbors, and co-workers increase a father's sense of well-being and encourage him to spend greater amounts of time with his child (Robins et al., 1981). Belsky (1979) postulates that men, lacking overt socialization for their fathering role, might be more influenced in the development of a parenting style by the nature of their social contacts than mothers. Similarly, Parke (n.d.) points to what he calls the greater "plasticity" of the father's role in infancy, the fact that the extent of a new father's interactions with his infant are considerably influenced both by the circumstances of the child's birth and the social supports for child-rearing he receives.

Other researchers, however, have found that mothering, too, is affected by variations in social networks and supports. Kessen and

Fein (1975) report that mothers who gained the most from home-based infant-education efforts were those who had the most extensive social networks. Several other studies have indicated that a high level of social contact with kin increases a mother's responsivity to her infant, which, in turn, has been correlated both with infant competence and a mother's enjoyment of her new maternal role (e.g., Bronfenbrenner, 1977; Feiring and Lewis, 1981; Unger and Powell, 1980). Crnic and associates (1981), reporting results of their study of 52 mother-premature infant pairs and 53 mother-full term infant pairs, have noted the importance of measuring mothers' satisfaction with the types of social supports available as well as the presence of support per se. They found that a mother's satisfaction with the amount and availability of her social supports (and not merely the presence or absence of such support) was a positive factor influencing the nature of mother-child interactions.

As a number of researchers point out, the confusion and disagreement over how social supports affect early parent-child interactions is in large part a reflection of the early stage of the research (Crnic et al., 1981; Cochran and Brassard, 1979; Dean and Lin, 1977; Mueller 1980). One major difficulty in trying to compare studies is that there are no set criteria (despite some extended discussions) for how to operationalize the terms "social supports" or "social network." Studies vary greatly in what they include and consider as social supports (from husband to extended kin to friends, neighbors, and professionals), in how crudely they measure the extent and availability of such supports, and in what populations are observed. Until further research is conducted and some consensus is reached, it will be difficult to advance our understanding of the evolution of the social worlds of new parents, or to assess accurately how differences in these social worlds affect the lives of the individuals involved—the mother, the father, and their new infant.

II. THE PRESCHOOL YEARS

Life with a preschooler reflects one of the many paradoxes involved in parenting: it at once constricts and expands a parent's social world. On the one hand, as the horizons of children expand beyond the confines of their homes, parents are pulled in new directions and into new involvements in the community in order to meet the needs and interests of their growing families. On the other hand, a preschooler's constant need for supervision and still limited abilities restrict a parent's options to move freely in a number of adult circles. The following section attempts to deal with both these aspects of parenting young children.

Unfortunately, as is the case for all stages of parenting, we have gathered more information on how children's developing skills and expanding social involvements affect the lives of mothers than on how they influence the daily activities and social interactions of fathers. There are a number of reasons for such a gender bias in the literature. First, women's lives continue to be most obviously reshaped by the presence of children; women, regardless of their employment status, continue to spend far more hours with their preschoolers than do men (e.g., Robinson, 1979; Walker and Woods, 1976). As the Newsons (1968) illustrate in their study of four-year-olds and their parents, preschoolers themselves often provide mothers with a major daily source of social intercourse and activity, and, at least in most cases, mothers truly enjoy the company of their increasing engaging child. A second factor accounting for the discrepancy in our knowledge of how parenting affects men's and women's lives is the return of a growing number of mothers to the paid labor force. In large part due to the economic costs of child-rearing, approximately two-fifths of all mothers with preschoolers (Presser, 1980) are currently employed, reflecting a trend which has generated considerable apprehension, interest, and research.

Also contributing to the lack of information on fathers of preschoolers is the fact that we are only starting to examine the place of fatherhood in contemporary men's lives. If, as Belsky (1979) and Parke (n.d.) suggest, peer support for active fathering increases a man's involvement in family life, the opposite is also true. As Lein (1979) describes, many men still are involved in social networks which tend to preserve traditional roles and continue to perceive paid work as their primary obligation to their young families. Work by Pleck (1979, 1980), however, indicates that these social roles may be in flux; men may be increasing their involvements in family life and household chores and may even be deriving greater satisfaction than in the past from their efforts.

At present, though, there are few studies which examine what being a father to a preschooler entails, and little discussion of how having a preschooler influences a father's social world. While fathers are mentioned in some research which examines the effects of social networks on such outcomes as preschoolers' verbal and social competence and maternal stress, they often are viewed not as primary members of the family in their own right (at least beyond being breadwinners and indicators of the family's social status), but as one of many members of the mother's support system (Rapoport et al., 1980). Research on fathering during the preschool years has a long way to go before it breaks out of the limited framework of the mother-child dyad.

One recent study which suggests that the effects of children on men's socal worlds are worth attention is the survey of 1,050 men and women residents of California conducted by Fischer and Oliker (1980). Results of this research indicate that the network size of men not only increases with marriage but continues to stay high during the time most men are parenting young children (that is, while they are under the age of 36). Kin, and not solely workmates and friends, are prominent members of men's social networks at this stage, perhaps a reflection of men's growing involvement in family life. Only after children are beyond preschool age is network size likely to decline. Research has also documented that young children bring men, as well as women, out into their neighborhoods; the early stages of child rearing coincide with both parents' most active participation in neighboring. As Stueve and Gerson (1977) report, "children play a strategic role in linking their parents to the neighborhood; they not only promote contacts with nearby parents but also curtail opportunities to interact socially away from home" (p. 85). In addition to providing parents and children with social opportunities, neighborhoods are relied on as sources of material and service exchanges. Clothes, toys, recreational equipment, child care, and the like are often exchanged among neighbors, thus reducing the total monetary costs of child rearing (e.g., Bane et al., 1979; Genovese, 1981).

Despite the opportunities which may be available in the neighborhood, however, many women remain socially constrained by their role as primary child-care provider. For instance, the extent of neighboring is dependent upon a number of variables, such as community size, neighborhood characteristics and history, and the demographic characteristics of women themselves (e.g., Bane, 1976; Keller, 1968; Michelson, 1977; Stimpson et al., 1980). If neighbors are not compatible, for example, women—especially those residing in suburban or rural areas—can find themselves isolated (e.g., Berger, 1960; Gans, 1967). Furthermore, as Saegert

(1981) points out, "distances to activities outside the home, lack of transportation and time schedules imposed by household duties and child care can leave women with little opportunity to expand their social lives outside the home and immediate neighborhood" (p. 97). In contrast to men, women's social network size declines after marriage and during the early child-rearing years (Fischer and Oliker, 1980). While women's networks are likely to expand again (after children are school-age and away from home for a good part of the day), this decline can result in a sense of loneliness and houseboundedness which continues beyond a child's infancy (e.g., Oakley, 1974; Rapoport et al., 1980). The social constraints imposed on women by young children (including a loss of leisure time to be enjoyed either alone or as part of a couple) may, at least in part, account for the fact that a number of surveys have found that parents at this stage of the child-rearing cycle are less likely to respond positively to questions about marital happiness than either childless couples anticipating parenthood or couples whose children are grown (Bane, 1976). Parents are not likely, however, to seek a divorce as a solution to their difficulties at this stage (Cherlin, 1978; Shaw, 1978). In a period where divorce is becoming increasingly acceptable as a way of dealing with marital unhappiness, this in part reflects the extent to which children cement even unhappy marital relations and in part the difficulties and expense of maintaining separate households when preschoolers are involved.

How a mother's return to the labor force effects the sense of constraint and possible isolation imposed by children is an interesting and as yet unanswered question. Clearly, taking a job reintroduces a woman to the social world of the workplace, and thus, by definition, often results in an increase in one aspect of her social network. Although most mothers of young children are employed for financial necessity, they point out that one of the most rewarding benefits of their jobs, after the salary, is that it gets them out of the house and brings them into contact with other adults (Cook, 1978). Employment, however, can also take time and energy away from other social involvements, particularly when a mother remains primarily responsible for both a young child and a home. Weiss et al.'s (1981) study of 151 white married mothers of three-year-olds indicates the complexity of the relationships between maternal employment and mothers' ability to maintain other forms of social contact. In their analyses, the investigators found that employment decreased the number of both total and functional (exchange-based) contacts among ethnic mothers while increasing contacts for non-ethnic mothers. While the research team postulates several reasons for this finding (e.g., employed ethnic mothers may concentrate their networks by relying on fewer people for different kinds of supports) the reasons for and implications of such a finding are still unclear. Unfortunately, this and similar research investigating the relationships among maternal employment, network size, level of informal support available to a family, and quality of family life is still in its earliest stages.

We do know, however, that social network members can be instrumental in meeting many of the needs of young families, whether or not a mother is employed. A number of national surveys have illustrated the importance of a family's social support system, both as a source of information about potential child-care possibilities and as a source of child care itself. With only approximately 5% of all children between the ages of three and five cared for in formal day-care centers, most families in which the mother is employed rely on informal sources of child-care support, be it spouses, other relatives, friends, or neighbors (Bane et al., 1979). Moreover, the social-support system provides child care whether mothers are employed or not. As the National Child Care Consumer Study (1975) illustrates, the vast majority of families use some form of non-parental child care, if only for occasional baby-sitting, and most families count on their social networks to provide such services.

To date, one bias of much of the research on networks and social supports is that it tends to take a family's network resources as a given. Few studies have addressed the question of how much work it takes to maintain the necessary informal support system so that it is available—for child care or for some other important service—when one needs it (an exception is work by Belle, 1981). It is generally agreed, however, that women remain primarily responsible for the unpaid work which is entailed in family-network building and maintenance (Bane, 1976). While some research suggests that women do not cut back this form of unpaid work when they take a paid job, the additional demands of employment can take a personal toll, such as the loss of sleep and personal time, which can be particularly severe when children are young. Bane et al. (1981) points out that the costs of maintaining an adequate social network to meet the needs for child care, social and leisure activity, and the like can be quite high and must be considered in terms of a wide spectrum of human costs. For example, what does grandmother expect in return for her child-care services, or how many hours must be paid back (and by whom) to the babysitting coop? We have only begun to recognize and examine the "paybacks" and unpaid labor which are involved in maintaining functioning social networks.

Labor is also required to ensure that young children receive what their parents view as important social and learning experiences. While the need for parents to search out appropriate formal activities for their children and to supervise their children's participation increases as children get older, a growing number of mothers and fathers begin scouting out and becoming involved in community-based children's programs while their offspring are still preschoolers. For example, although as recently as 1967 only 6.8% of the nation's three-year-olds were enrolled in preschools, by 1976 this figure had increased to 20%. Over 80% of all five-year-olds currently attend some form of preschool program, and both public and private provision of nursery and kindergarten programs has increased dramatically during this same period (Bane et al., 1980). The ramifications of these figures on the social worlds of parents are far-reaching.

First, these early school encounters introduce parents to a new world of child-serving professionals. As the Newsons (1968) illustrate, school entry is a major marker in the life of the family—it is the first major contact of a child with an outside and often judgmental institution. Parents prepare children for this day by stepping up the pace of their child's social activity; they also often become anxious about how their child will be judged by the standards of outsiders and about whether the values and child-rearing styles of the preschool teachers are similar to their own (e.g., Joffe, 1977). In addition, preschool programs provide parents with the opportunity to meet other parents with children the same age. The importance of such contacts has been documented in the case of Headstart. A number of evaluations of Headstart programs have shown that one of the most positive and long-term outcomes of children's participation is the opportunity parents have to meet other parents in informal support groups (e.g., Lazar et al., 1977). Often, the friends made through Headstart and other preschool programs become important sources of social support, particularly for women, for many years after children have moved on to new situations. Many preschool programs and activities like Headstart encourage (if not actively require) parent participation. The volunteer time spent in such organizations often marks the beginning of parents' increased formal involvements in their communities. Participation in programs for young children serve as a stepping stone to later participation in more formal school-based PTAs, sports teams, children's organizations, and the like.

Perhaps most importantly, these types of early interactions with child-serving institutions serve as reminders of the fact that preschoolers do not merely constrain their parents' social lives. Young children also bring parents out into their neighborhoods and communities and integrate them into new forms of social involvements. Such involvements increase a family's sense of local attachment and add a new layer to men's and women's social worlds. In doing so, they also provide the community with ways of monitoring and influencing an individual family's child-rearing efforts, successes, and failures. Through these outside encounters, the presence of children gradually forces parents to reshape their notions of the interface between the private world of the family and the public world of the community at large.

III. THE SCHOOL YEARS

Although most girls and boys have attended some preschool program for one or more years before they are officially enrolled in kindergarten or first grade, the transition from the generally small and comparatively informal preschool environment to the more formal and bureaucratized world of the public school requires many adjustments, for both parents and their children. As the authors of *Crestwood Heights* point out:

> The nursery school teacher advises the parents on child-rearing problems, but it does not lie in her power to "pass" or "fail" the child . . . instead of being a partner in responsibility, as was the case with the nursery school child, the parent assumes a far smaller role in the educational enterprise of the public school. (Seeley et al., 1956, p. 96)

Moreover, in addition to involvement with school, the school-aged child also becomes increasingly engaged in a number of other neighborhood and community activities, from after-school play with peers to participation in scouting, sports teams, and church activities. No longer are children under maternal supervision for most of the day; both mothers and children find new ways to spend their time as schools and other community-based organizations replace the need for parents to provide the bulk of child care and social and educational instruction.

Despite the growing independence of children and parents at this stage, there are many ways in which their social lives continue to be intricately entwined. First, mothers and fathers do not just hand over their children to child-serving institutions. Most take seriously their responsibility to monitor children's interactions with the outside world. Parents, acting on their own values, take an active role in integrating their children into the community and mediating between the outside world and their own family (O'Donnell and Stueve, forthcoming).

Furthermore, schools and extracurricular activities, while clearly providing supports for child-rearing, do not totally supplant the role of parents as child-care providers. Once again, the most obvious example of how concern for the needs of children continues to shape their parents' social interactions is the way most mothers base their decisions of whether to take a paid job, the hours of their employment, and even the location of their jobs around child-rearing responsibilities. Although slightly over one-half of all mothers of school-aged children are currently in the labor force, a number of studies indicate that both working- and middle-class mothers try to restrict paid-work hours so that they can limit the conflict between their employment and family roles (e.g., Cook, 1978; Hayghe, 1980; O'Donnell and Stueve, 1981; Schoenberg, 1980). Usually, researchers talk of these employment decisions in terms of constraints—part-time hours clearly limit a woman's status and upward mobility in the workplace. Mothers also mention the positive aspects of part-time hours; not only does part-time work lessen some of the stresses of paid employment, but it also provides an employed mother with the advantages of social contacts at the workplace and the opportunity to engage in what many regard as an important and enjoyable social contact with their children when they arrive home from school (Friedland and Kort, 1981; O'Donnell and Stueve, forthcoming).

The demands (and pleasures) of child rearing influence more than just mothers' work schedules. A recent study of eighty white mothers residing in a mixed working- and middle-class suburb found that almost four times as many of the employed mothers worked right in the community in which they lived as did employed fathers (O'Donnell and Stueve, 1981). Mothers did so in order to cut down the time and energy costs of commuting and to ensure that they would be readily available if some emergency arose and their children needed them. Moreover, maternal employment in the community appeared to increase other forms of local involvement. Neighbors were likely to be the source of information about job possibilities and child care arrangements; they were also likely to be co-workers and occasional babysitters. In light of these findings, the researchers argue that instead of becoming less salient to the lives of families, the local community may actually be increasing in importance—it is now looked to as a source of women's jobs which are close to home and school.

Both employed and unemployed mothers of school-aged children continue to spend considerable amounts of time in neighboring and continue to participate in a wide variety of neighborhood and community-based activities. For example, the fact that women circumscribe their paid-work hours around the needs of children (and many remain full-time homemakers) does not mean that they remain in their homes. There is evidence that mothers make great efforts to participate in a variety of community-based activities, whether they do so by limiting their employment or subtracting hours from their own personal and leisure time. Mothers have maintained a tradition of participation in church, school, and other voluntary organizations, particularly those which sponsor children's programs. While there are reported differences across social-class groups, with middle-class women more likely to spend a greater number of hours volunteering, the presence of children continues to pull a great number of mothers into unpaid community work (Coser, 1964; Hybels, 1978; O'Donnell and Stueve, forthcoming; Schoenberg, 1981). Despite disclaimers from some feminists that this type of unpaid work is exploitative of women and the fact that an increasing proportion of mothers are now working at paid jobs, many women continue to see volunteer work as an important aspect of their roles as wives and mothers, much as they did almost twenty years ago. At that time, Coser (1964) stated that along with the choice of a neighborhood, a mother's work with community organizations is "another at least equally important means of integration between the values governing the family and those governing the community. . . . Through her activities in the PTA, Brownies, cub scouts, and the like, she helps both to maintain the communal social network and to integrate her children in it'' (p. 377; see also LeMasters, 1970). Bane (1976) suggests that the work mothers perform for child-serving organizations provides women with ''a formal structure for social activity that can supplement the informal network of visiting and shared activity with friends and neighbors'' (p. 62). In addition, it provides families with a means of retaining some level of supervision over their children's involvements in the community. Work with schools and community-based children's organizations is recognized by parents as a productive way of monitoring both children's progress and the mannerisms and values of the professionals their families come into contact with.

A number of post-war community studies illustrated how much of a role women have played in community building through their unpaid work. They also indicated how much of a time and energy drain this work often entails (Gans, 1967; Seeley et al., 1956). Whether women now have either as much time to devote to such activities or as much of a commitment has been open to question. A few recent studies have investigated the relationship between maternal paid employment and volunteer work and found that employed mothers with school-aged children often retain a commitment to volunteer-community work, although women stress that their involvement is related to their stage in the child-rearing process and that it will decrease as children get older (O'Donnell and Stueve, forthcoming; Rubin and Medrich, 1980; Schoenberg, 1980). In fact, Schoenberg (1980) suggests that employment may be narrowing some of the class distinctions previously documented. Rather than decreasing a working-class woman's level of volunteer participation, she found that employment seemed to increase involvement. Whereas working-class women have been characterized as more likely to restrict their social interactions to kin and the immediate neighborhood, with only occasional forays into the middle-class world of volunteer work, her study suggests that the skills and increased sense of comfort with institutions working-class women obtain from paid jobs may actually increase their desire to participate in volunteer organizations. Whereas the traditional model looks at volunteer work as a stepping-stone to paid employment (Hybels, 1978; Loeser, 1974), this interesting small-scale study suggests that there may be ways that paid work also acts as a training ground for greater community participation.

While research illustrates how children's engagements in a number of activities outside the home act both as incentives and catalysts for their mothers' involvements in the wider community, there is little documentation of the connections between the demands of fathering and men's community participation. While the existence of Little League teams and boy-scout troops serve as testimony to fathers' involvements, we know little about the extent of or variations in men's participation in child-serving institutions, beyond the fact that parenting also appears to pull men, although to a lesser degree than women, into unpaid community work (Hybels, 1978). In part, our lack of knowledge is due to the fact that volunteer work and this aspect of community building has most often been conceptualized (if it is thought of at all) as an aspect of women's work. In years past, community studies emphasized the limited role fathers played in such organizations, and most researchers and theorists have continued to view the mother as the critical link between the family and child-serving institutions (e.g., Donzelot, 1980; Hollingshead, 1945; Lightfoot, 1978; Seeley et al., 1956).

Whether there have been any changes in this aspect of fathering over the past several decades is unclear—for example, does a wife's employment affect her husband's volunteer participation? There is some research to indicate that men may be retaining their secondary role, particularly in school-related parents' groups (Joffe, 1977; Lightfoot, 1978; O'Donnell and Stueve, forthcoming; Steinberg, 1980). Even though many of the women interviewed in Steinberg's (1980) study of grass roots participation were employed, they continued to attend more meetings and have higher levels of participation in school-parent groups than their spouses. Steinberg states that the major change in fathers' participation over the past several decades may be that today more men are "willing" to let their wives attend meetings and to babysit in their absence. As a result, she suggests that women may not only be continuing their unpaid work, but, with the rise of both feminism and concern with community participation, may actually be increasing the power and influence they exert over some community institutions, such as the schools. Furthermore, Steinberg's research reminds us that we must view a mother's participation in volunteer work in the context of her broader participation in neighborhood and community life. A mother's ability to mobilize support and build a power base was found to be related to the extent of her social network, her "preexisting social ties and access to opportunities to interact with other mothers at the community level" (p. 237). Not surprisingly, given what we know about the nature of a mother's social world, these ties are most likely to be formed through women's involvements in child-related activities, through schools, community organizations, neighborhoods, and a variety of recreational facilities.

Unfortunately, we are nowhere near this level of investigation or understanding in regards to how children influence the social and community involvements of their fathers. How much of our ignorance is a reflection of a gender bias in available research and how much is an accurate reflection of the differential impact of school-aged children on the lives of women and men is unclear. It is possible that fathers of school-aged children, caught in the life-cycle squeeze which demands that they earn more money as children grow older and the costs of maintaining a family rise, put most of their energy into their breadwinning role and leave much of the unpaid work entailed in neighborhood and community building to their wives. However, in light of the continued and obvious involvement of men in some levels of neighborhood and community life (from exchanging tools with the people who live next door to participating in a variety of church and civic organizations) more research is clearly needed on fathers' child-rearing activities. A new generation of fathers who are accustomed to the idea of their wives' employment, who are becoming more involved with their children's births and early years, and who are looking to their families for greater sources of satisfaction and support may well find it necessary to increase their involvements in other aspects of child-rearing as well. This increased involvement could include such activities as attending parent-teacher conferences and donating more time to child-serving institutions. If so, fathers may find that their lives and social worlds are being shaped by children in ways beyond their expectations. It is also possible, however, that the added stresses and demands of their wives' employment and fathers' increasing participation in family life may actually decrease the amount of time men have available for unpaid community work. Which avenue is taken may depend on whether men find community work, from neighboring to coaching a sports team, enjoyable and rewarding. Men appear to take on the pleasurable tasks associated with child-rearing, such as reading stories and putting children to bed before they share in some of the more onerous duties, such as cleaning the bathroom, shuffling children to doctor appointments, and the like (Lein, 1980). Whatever the case, there is clearly a need for additional research which documents the connections and intersections between the paid and unpaid work of men and women, and the impact of a family's division of unpaid and paid labor on the social worlds of both mothers and fathers.

CONCLUSION

In assessing the evidence on how children affect the social worlds of mothers and fathers, it is striking to note both the diversity of ways and the extent to which children shape the informal relations and more formal ties of their parents. What has emerged in the preceding discussion is an account of how being a parent not only shapes one's personal life and interactions, but how parenthood influences and often strengthens an adult's connections to extended family, neighbors, friends, and the larger community. Far too often, we think of parenting in the most limited terms—basic child care, domestic chores, and income provision. Yet raising children in modern society clearly involves far more. Making arrangements so that grandparents and children will have time together, taking care to meet and choose a babysitter who will best fit one's needs and values, finding out about children's activities offered in the community, meeting with teachers and the other professionals who work with family members, attending PTA meetings, serving as scout leaders and sports coaches, and so on may all be a part of the fabric of every day family life, but, as separate tasks and activities, they are too often ignored, particularly in discussions of the work entailed in child-rearing and the stresses and satisfaction of being a parent.

In addition to bringing to the forefront some of these more subtle and often neglected aspects of parenting, one further issue warrants attention, both in terms of how we think about what it means to be a parent and in terms of how we frame future research. In part because this review primarily examined a unidirectional process, that is, children's influence on parents (and, in particular, how children differentially influence the social relations of men and women) and, in part, because of the limitations of previous research, much of the work reported here leaves us with the inaccurate impression that the social worlds of individuals within a family—mother, father, and child—are more conceptually discrete and bounded than, in reality, they are. We have only begun to take the first steps towards understanding how nuclear-family members operate as "a system of reciprocal and interacting influences" (Parke and Savin, 1980, p. 46). We have far to go before we understand the ways in which the social worlds of individuals within a family, including both the intimate relations among household members and their connections with a variety of people and institutions outside the nuclear family, are also reciprocal and interacting. In the future, it will be important to explore the complexities and intricate connections among the social worlds of parents and children. For example, we still have much to learn about the interactions among such factors as husbands' employment schedule and work commitments, wives' employment decisions and work patterns, parents' participation in children's activities and community-based, child-serving institutions, and children's involvements in community life. What we need now is not only more research which investigates the impact of parenting and the parenting career on men's and women's lives as individuals, but also work which conceptualizes and investigates the intersecting and overlapping social worlds of parents and children. By using such a framework, it may be possible to develop the construct of "the social worlds of families" and to come to a greater understanding of differences in how families, taken as systems, relate to and interact with the world outside the home.

REFERENCES

Bane, M. J. *Here to stay.* New York: Basic Books, 1976.

Bane, M. J., Lein, L., O'Donnell, L., and Stueve, A. The costs of child care. *Working Mother*, February 1981.

Bane, M. J., Lein, L., O'Donnell L., Stueve, A., and Welles, B. Child care arrangements of working parents. *Monthly Labor Review*, October 1979, *102*, 50–55.

Bell, R. Q. A reinterpretation of the direction of effects in studies of socialization. *Psychological Review*, 1968, *75*, 81–95.

Bell, R. Q., and Harper, L. V. *Child effects on adults.* Hillsdale, N.J.: L. Erlbaum Associates, 1977.

Belle, D. The social network as a source of both stress and support to low-income mothers. Paper presented at the Biennial Meeting of the Society for Research on Child Development, Boston, April 1981.

Belsky, J. The interrelation of parental and spousal behavior during infancy in traditional nuclear families: An exploratory analysis. *Journal of Marriage and the Family*, 1979, *41*, 749–755.

Berger, B. *Working class suburb.* Berkeley: University of California Press, 1960.

Bernard, J. *The future of motherhood.* New York: Penguin Books, 1974.

Bott, E. *Family and social networks*. London: Tavistock Publications, 1957.

Bronfenbrenner, U. Toward an experimental ecology of human development. *American Psychologist*, 1977, *32*, 513–531.

Brown, G. W. *Social origins of depression: A study of psychiatric disorder in women*. New York: Free Press, 1974.

Campbell, A., Converse, P. E., and Rogers, W. L. *The quality of American life*. New York: Russell Sage Foundation, 1976.

Cherlin, A. Employment, income, and family life: The case of marital dissolution. In *Women's changing roles at home and on the job, a special report of the National Commission for Manpower Policy*, No. 26., September 1978.

Cochran, M. M., and Brassard, J. A. Child development and parental social networks. *Child Development*, 1979, *50*, 601–616.

Cook, A. *The working mother*. Ithaca, N.Y.: Cornell University, 1978.

Coser, R. Authority and structural ambivalence in the middle-class family. In R. Coser (Ed.), *The family, its structure and function*. New York: St. Martins Press, 1964.

Cowan, C. P., and Cowan, P. A. Couple role arrangements and satisfaction during family formation. Paper presented at the Biennial Meeting of the Society for Research in Child Development, Boston, April 1981.

Cowan, C. P., Cowan, P. A., Coie, L., and Coie, J. D. Becoming a family: The impact of a first child's birth on the couple's relationship. In W. B. Miller and L. F. Newman (Eds.), *The first child and family formation*. Chapel Hill: Carolina Population Center, University of North Carolina, 1978.

Crnic, K. A., Greenberg, M. T., Ragozin, A. S., Robinson, N. M., and Basham, R. The effects of stress and social support on maternal attitudes and the mother infant relationship. Paper presented at the Biennial Meeting of the Society for Research in Child Development, Boston, April 1981.

Dean, A., and Lin, N. The stress buffering role of social support. *Journal of Nervous and Mental Diseases*, 1977, *165*, 403–417.

Donzelot, J. *The policing of families*. New York: Pantheon Books, 1979.

Dyer, E. D. Parenthood as crisis: A restudy. *Marriage and Family Living*, May 25, 1963, 196–201.

Entwisle, D. R. Preparation for childbirth and parenting. In *Families Today*, v.1, Washington, D.C.: National Institute of Mental Health Science Monograph, Stock Number 017–024–00955–5, 1979, 143–171.

Entwisle, D. R., and Doering, S. G. *The first birth*. Baltimore: The Johns Hopkins Univeristy Press, 1980.

Featherstone, H. *A difference in the family*. New York: Basic Books, 1980.

Fein, R. A. Men's experiences before and after the birth of a first child: Dependence, marital sharing, and anxiety. Unpublished doctoral dissertation, Harvard University, 1974.

Feiring, C. G., and Lewis, W. The social networks of three year old children. Paper presented at the Biennial Meeting of the Society for Research in Child Development, Boston, April 1981.

Fischer, C. S. *The urban experience*. New York: Harcourt Brace Jovanovich Inc., 1976.

Fischer, C., Jackson, R. M., Stueve, C. A., Gerson, K., Jones, L. M., with Baldassare, M. *Networks and places*. New York: Free Press, 1977.

Fischer, C., and Oliker, M. Friendships, sex, and the life cycle. Working paper, University of California, Berkeley: Institute of Urban and Regional Development, 1980.

Fried, M. *The world of the urban working class*. Cambridge: Harvard University Press, 1973.

Friedland, R., and Kort, C. *The mother's book, shared experiences*. Boston: Houghton Mifflin Company, 1981.

Gans, H. *The Levittowners*. New York: Pantheon, 1967.

Genovese, R. G. A women's self-help network as a response to service needs in the suburbs. In C. R. Stimpson, E. Dixler, M. J. Nelson, and K. B. Yatrakis (Eds.), *Women and the American city*. Chicago: University of Chicago Press, 1980.

Gilstrap, B. J., Pfeiffenberger, C., and Belsky, J. Psychological preparation for parenthood and its relation to parental and marital behavior: An exploratory analysis. Paper presented at the Biennial Meeting of the Society for Research on Child Development, Boston, April 1981.

Glenn, N. D. Psychological well-being in the postparental stage: Some evidence from national surveys. *Journal of Marriage and the Family,* 1975, *37,* 105–110.

Glenn, N. D., and Weaver, C. N. A multisurvey of marital happiness. *Journal of Marriage and the Family, 40,* 1978, 269–282.

Gold, C., and Gold, E. J. *Joyous childbirth.* New York: Signet Books, 1977.

Grossman, F. K., Eichler, L. S., and Winickoff, S. A. *Pregnancy, birth, and parenthood.* San Francisco: Jossey-Bass Publishers, 1980.

Hall, R. E. *Nine months reading.* New York: Bantam Books, 1972.

Hayghe, H. Marital and family characteristics of workers—March 1977. *Monthly Labor Review,* February 1978, 51–54.

Hill, R. *Family development in three generations: A longitudinal study of changing family patterns of planning and achievement.* Cambridge: Schenkman, 1970.

Hobbs, D. Transition to parenthood, a replication and an extension. *Journal of Marriage and the Family,* 1968, *30,* 413–417.

Hobbs, D. F., Jr., and Cole, S. P. Transition to parenthood: A decade replication. *Journal of Marriage and the Family,* 1976, *38,* 723–731.

Hoffman, L. W. Effects of a first child on women's social role development. In W. B. Miller and L. Newman (Eds.), *The first child and family formation.* Chapel Hill: Carolina Population Center, 1978.

Hoffman, L. W., and Manis, J. D. Influences of children on marital interaction and parental satisfaction and dissatisfaction. In R. M. Lerner and G. B. Spanier (Eds.), *Child influences on marital and family interaction: A life-span perspective.* New York: Academic Press, 1978.

Hollingshead, A. B. *Elmstown youth and Elmstown revisited.* New York: John Wiley and Sons, 1945 and 1975.

Hybels, J. H. Volunteer jobs to paid jobs: A study of the transition. Report to the ACTION agency under contract number 78–043–1008, May 1978.

Joffe, C. E. *Friendly intruders, child care, professionals, and family life.* Berkeley: University of California Press, 1977.

Keller, S. *The urban neighborhood.* New York: Random House, 1968.

Kessen, W., and Fein, G. *Volunteers in home-based infant education: Language, play and social development.* Final report to the Office of Child Development of the Department of Health, Education, and Welfare, August 1975.

La Rossa, R., and LaRossa, M. M. *Transition to parenthood: How infants change families.* Beverly Hills: Sage Publications, 1981.

Lazar, I., Hubbell, V. R., Murray, H., Rosche, M. B., and Royce, J. *The persistence of preschool effects.* Final report to the Administration on Children, Youth and Families, U.S. Department of Health, Education, and Welfare, October 1977. (DHEW Pub. No. OHDS 78–30129)

Lein, L. Male participation in home life: Impact of social supports and breadwinner responsibility on the allocation of tasks. *Family Coordinator,* October 1979, 489–495.

LeMasters, E. Parenthood as crises. *Marriage and Family Living,* 1957, *19,* 352–355.

LeMasters, E. *Parents in modern America.* Homeward, Ill.: Dorsey Press, 1970.

Lerner, R. M., and Spanier, G. B. (Eds.) *Child influences on marital and family interaction.* New York: Academic Press, 1978.

Lewis, M., and Rosenblum, L. (Eds.) *The effect of the infant on its caregiver.* New York: John Wiley & Sons, 1974.

Lewis, M., and Weinraub, M. The father's role in the child's social network. In Lamb, M. (Ed.), *The role of the father in child development.* New York: John Wiley & Sons, 1976.

Lightfoot, S. L. *Worlds apart: Relationships between families and schools.* New York: Basic Books, 1978.

Loeser, H. *Women, work, and volunteering.* Boston: Beacon Press, 1974.

Lopata, H. Z. *Occupation housewife.* New York: Oxford University Press, 1971.

Meyerowitz, J. H., and Feldman, H. Transitions to parenthood. *Psychiatric Research Report,* 1966, *20,* 78–84.

Michelson, W. *Environmental choice, human behavior, and residential satisfaction.* New York: Oxford University Press, 1977.

Mueller, D. P. Social network: A promising direction for research on the relationship of the social environment to psychiatric disorders. *Social Science and Medicine,* 1980, *14a,* 147–161.

Newson, J., and Newson, E. *Four years old in an urban community.* Chicago: Aldine Atheston, 1968.

Oakley, A. *Becoming a mother.* New York: Schocken Books, 1980.

Oakley, A. *Housewife.* London: Allen Lane, 1974.

O'Donnell, L. N., and Stueve, A. Mothers as social agents: Integrating children into the community. In H. Z. Lopata and J. Pleck (Eds.), *Research in interweave of social roles,* V. II, forthcoming.

O'Donnell, L. N., and Stueve, A. Employed women: Mothers and good neighbors. *The urban and social change review, special issue on neighborhood and community,* Winter 1981, *14,* 21–26.

Oppenheimer, V. K. The life-cycle squeeze: The interaction of men's occupational and family life cycles. *Demography,* May 1974, *11,* 227–245.

Osofsky, J. D., and O'Connell, E. L. Parent-child interaction. *Developmental Psychology,* 1972, *7*(2), 157–168.

Parke, R. D. The father-infant relationship: A family perspective. To appear in P. Berman (Ed.), *Women: A developmental perspective,* n.d.

Parke, R. D., and O'Leary, S. Father-mother-infant interaction in the newborn period: Some findings, some observations, and some unresolved issues. In K. Riegel and J. Meacham (Eds.), *The Developing Individual in a Changing World,* v. 2, *Social and Environmental Issues.* The Hague: Mouton, 1975.

Peterson, G. H., and Mehl, L. E. Comparative studies of psychological outcome of various childbirth alternatives. In L. Stewart and D. Stewart (Eds.), *21st Century obstetrics now.* Chapel Hill: NAPSAC, 1977.

Pleck, J. Men's family work: Three perspectives and some new data. *The Family Coordinator,* 1979, *26,* 481–488.

Pleck, J., Staines, G., and Lang, L. Work and family life: First reports on work-family interference and workers' formal child care arrangements, from the 1977 Quality of Employment Survey. Working Paper No. 63, Wellesley College Center for Research on Women, 1978.

Presser, H. Working women and child care. Paper presented at the Research Conference on Women: A Developmental Perspective, sponsored by the National Institute on Child Health and Human Development in cooperation with the National Institute of Mental Health and the National Institute of Aging, November 1980.

Rapoport, R., Rapoport, R. N., Strelitz, Z., with Kew, S. *Fathers, mothers, and society.* New York: Vintage Books, 1977.

Raush, H. L., Barry, W. A., Herterl, R. K., and Swain, M. A. *Communication, conflict, and marriage.* San Francisco: Jossey-Bass, 1974.

Robins, E., Gamble, W., and Belsky, J. The wider ecology of infancy. Paper presented at the Biennial Meeting of the Society for Research in Child Development, Boston, April 1981.

Robinson, J. *How Americans use time.* New York: Praeger, 1977.

Rodes, T. W., and Moore, J. C. National child care consumer study, Vol. 3. Arlington, Va.: Unco, Inc., 1975.

Rollins, B., and Feldman, H. Marital satisfaction over the family life cycle. *Journal of Marriage and the Family*, 1970, *32*, 20–28.

Rossi, A. Transition to parenthood. *Journal of Marriage and the Family*, 1968, *30*, 26–39.

Rubin, L. *Worlds of pain*. New York: Basic Books, 1976.

Rubin, V., and Medrick, E. Child care, recreation, and the fiscal crisis. *The Urban and Social Change Review*, 1979, *12*, 22–26.

Russell, C. Transition to parenthood: Problems and gratifications. *Journal of Marriage and the Family*, 1974, *36*, 294–301.

Saegert, S. Masculine cities and feminine suburbs: Polarized ideas, contradictory realities. In C. R. Stimpson, E. Dixler, M. J. Nelson, and K. B. Yatrakis (Eds.), *Women and the American city*. Chicago: University of Chicago Press, 1980.

Schvaneveldt, J. D., and Ihinger, M. Sibling relations in the family. In W. R. Burr, R. Hill, F. Nye, and I. Neiss (Eds.), *Contemporary theories about the family*. New York: Free Press, 1979, 453–467.

Schoenberg, S. P. Some trends in the community: Participation of women in their neighborhoods. In C. R. Stimpson, E. Dixler, M. J. Nelson, and K. B. Yatrakis (Eds.), *Women and the American city*. Chicago: University of Chicago Press, 1980.

Seeley, J. R., Sim, R. A., and Loosley, E. W. *Crestwood Heights*. Toronto: University of Toronto Press, 1956.

Shapiro, D., and Mott, F. L. Labor supply behavior of prospective and new mothers. *Demography*, 1979, *16*, 199–208.

Shaw, L. B. Economic consequences of marital disruption. In *Women's changing roles at home and on the job*. A special report of the National Commission for Manpower Policy, No. 26, September 1978.

Slater, P. Social limitations on libidinal withdrawal. In R. L. Coser, (Ed.), *The family: Its structure and functions*. New York: St. Martins Press, 1964.

Sokoloff, N. *Between money and love: The dialectics of women's home and market work*. New York: Praeger Publishers, 1980.

Steinberg, L. S. The role of women's social networks in the adoption of innovation at the grass-roots level. In C. R. Stimpson, E. Dixler, M. J. Nelson, and K. B. Yatrakis (Eds.), *Women and the American city*. Chicago: University of Chicago Press, 1980.

Stueve, C. A., and Gerson, K. Personal relations across the life-cycle. In C. Fischer et al. (Eds.), *Networks and places*. New York: Free Press, 1977, 79–100.

Sussman, M. Relationships of adult children with their parents in the United States. In E. Shanas and G. Strieb (Eds.), *Social structure and the family*. Englewood Cliffs, N.J.: Prentice-Hall, 1965.

Unger, D., and Powell, D. Supporting families under stress: The role of social networks. *Family Relations*, 1980, *29*, 566–574.

U.S. Department of Labor. *Dual careers. A longitudinal study of labor market experience of workers*. Manpower Research Monograph No. 21, v. 2, Washington, D.C.: U.S. Government Printing Office, 1973.

U.S. Department of Labor. *Young workers and their families*. Special Labor Force Report, 233, October 1979.

Walker, K., and Woods, M. E. *Time use: A measure of household production of family goods and services*. Washington, D.C.: American Home Economics Association, 1976.

Weiss, H., Henderson, C., Jr., Campbell, M., and Cochran, M. The effects of informal social networks or mothers' perceptions of themselves as parents: A preliminary report. Paper presented at the Biennial Meeting of the Society for Research on Child Development, April 1981.

Yarrow, M. R., Waxler, C. A., and Scott, P. M. Child effects on adult behavior. *Developmental Psychology*, 1971, *5*(2), 300–311.

Young, M., and Willmott, P. *Family and kinship in East London*. London: Routledge and Kegan Paul, 1957.

The Social-Support Systems
of Black Families

Michelene Malson

INTRODUCTION

Since kin-support systems were recognized by Robert Hill in 1971 as one of the main sources of strength in Black families, discussion and inquiry about them have been a central theme in Black family studies. In fact, social-support systems consisting of kin, friends, and neighbors have become a focal point of studies of families on the whole, although there is still disagreement over their definition and their component parts.

This paper will review contemporary literature on Black families' social-support systems, using a broad definition of social-support systems as "a set of personal contacts through which the individual maintains his social identity and receives emotional supports, material aid and services, information and new social contacts" (Walker et al., 1977).[1] First, this review takes a theoretical perspective. It is unclear whether variables used to describe social-support systems in general, i.e., network composition and durability, have also been used or are applicable to describe social-support systems of Black families. Second, the review will describe the empirical work done on Black families' social-support systems, assess our knowledge about these systems in different kinds of Black families, and identify the areas where more empirical work on this topic is needed.

Black families have historically been involved in support systems, particularly those that connect extended kin. Frazier (1939), in one of the earliest examinations of Black families, described the

Michelene Malson is Program Director for the Minority Women's Program at the Wellesley College Center for Research on Women.

extended family in the rural South. In *Black Families in Slavery and Freedom* (1976), Gutman presented evidence of the presence of Black family support systems on slave plantations in the South. The functions that they provided included those they still provide today, such as the informal adoption of members who were often unrelated. Pleck (1980) described the mutual support systems of Black families in 19th-century Boston. Historically, Black kin and friends have been instrumental in providing aid and in-kind services for Black families and children who have been systematically excluded from the formal social service system (Billingsley and Giovannoni, 1971).

While Black social-support systems have long existed, recognition of their role in Black family functioning may not have occurred without other theoretical developments in Black family studies. Allen (1978) summarized three theoretical positions that have been used to examine Black families. The "cultural equivalent" perspective assumes that Black families have cultures similar to those of white families. Therefore, Black families are easily compared with white families. The "cultural deviant" model views Black families as aberrations of middle-class white families. This model suggests that the cultural differences found in Black families are deviations from normalcy represented by middle-class white families and therefore pathological. The "cultural variant" perspective sees the differences in Black family form and structure as strengths in their social structure instead of weaknesses. Where differences are either denied or viewed as abnormal in the first two models, the "cultural variant" model views them as sensible adaptations to external stresses and forces. This model interprets variations in role behavior and functioning as attempts to function under extreme economic and social conditions (Billingsley, 1968).

The contemporary literature on Black families' social-support systems has developed as an extension of the cultural variant perspective on Black families. This theoretical perspective views the mutual aid and emotional support exchanged by members of the support system as a strength of the social system. Within this conceptual framework, the support systems of Black families are seen as a constructive adaptation.

Using the cultural variant perspective, this article will try to delineate the specific characteristics and functions of social-support systems surrounding different kinds of Black families. It examines the hypothesis that social-support systems are a strength of

Black families, providing needed aid and services that help insure family functioning.

METHODOLOGIES USED TO STUDY
THE SOCIAL-SUPPORT SYSTEMS OF BLACK FAMILIES

Methods used for the empirical investigation of the social-support systems of Black families include both ethnographic and social survey procedures. Within these two broad categories, researchers have used different data collection procedures and resources, sample sizes, and analytic methods, and they have collected data on Black families in various sites in the United States.

1. Ethnographic Approach

The purpose of the ethnographic approach is to provide a detailed descriptive account of the processes and interworkings of family life. This approach is most often associated with Stack's 1974 study of the kin and mutual-aid systems of Black families in a midwestern urban site. Those employing this perspective often investigate families in one community (Stack, 1973, 1974; Ashenbrenner, 1973, 1975), although Martin and Martin (1978) investigated families in four sites, including rural and urban communities. The ethnographic data collection procedure usually includes participant observation done over time. In Stack's case she became an observer and often a participant for a number of years in the mutual exchange systems she described. The Martins studied their sample families from 1969–1977.

Besides undertaking participant observation, ethnographers conduct unstructured and informal interviews, and often group interviews (Martin and Martin, 1978). Genealogical trees and family histories are frequently a data collection technique. In addition, Stack (1974) used quantitative data sources such as AFDC records on recipiency rates and living arrangements of dependent children.

One of the criticisms of the ethnographic approach is the small sample size. While she studied others, Stack's main hypotheses and observations were based primarily on in-depth analysis of the kin-help and mutual systems of the two families, the Jacksons and the Waters. However, it might be argued that the sample sizes used in the ethnographic approach are actually larger than they appear since extended families tend to be composed of many members. Martin and Martin (1978) studied 30 extended families and as many as 20 "key" members in each; they reported that some extended families had as many as 100. The families and key members studied included more than a thousand persons.

2. Social Survey Approach

Little attention had been placed on the use of large scale social surveys to examine the characteristics of Black families' social-support systems prior to Robert Hill's work of the 70s. *The Strengths of Black Families* (1972) and *Informal Adoption Among Black Families* (1977) were some of the first studies employing secondary analyses of large scale data to describe Black family kin systems. For instance, Hill (1977) used data from the decennial Census, Bureau of the Census Current Population Surveys, and a Public Use Sample to describe national trends in extended Black families and informal adoption as well as their economic and social characteristics. Allen (1979) also used census materials to describe the association between extended family structure, household living arrangements, and income.[2]

Other social surveys use smaller samples, usually 300 or less, and more extensive instruments, to study Black families' support systems. This type of survey is exemplified by the work of McAdoo. Sites for her studies are usually urban (1981) and/or suburban (1978), mid-Atlantic locales. Approximately 300 respondents were interviewed in both studies. In one, persons seen as significant contributors to individuals' social networks were also interviewed. Data were collected in the 1978 study using the McAdoo Family Profile Scale which was developed because no existing instrument had been developed to assess social networks and mobility in Black families.

McAdoo's work has had great impact on the study of Black families' social-support systems. First, it has consistently emphasized the importance of social-support systems as a strategic variable in the functioning of Black families. Second, her work not only describes the nature and characteristics of social-support systems and mutual exchange but goes further to investigate the relationship between these and other variables such as social and economic mobility (1978) and stress (1981).

THE CHARACTERISTICS AND PURPOSES
OF SOCIAL-SUPPORT SYSTEMS

One shortcoming of the research on the support systems of Black families is the lack of a systematic investigation of the theoretical assumptions underlying participation in them. These systems, like social-support systems in other families, can be described in terms of those who participate, the assumptions underlying their participation, and the tasks the system accomplishes.

1. System Composition and Social Ties

In fact, Black families may form relationships with kin, friends, or neighbors. Although most social interaction of Black families is reportedly with kin, interaction with others has not been given serious investigation.

a. Kin. Studies report that the frequency of interaction with kin is dependent upon their proximity, with the highest degree occurring when kin live in the same neighborhood or city. Because of limited mobility among Black families, geographical proximity leads to support systems that are primarily kin-centered (Martineau, 1977; McAdoo, 1978; Hays and Mindel, 1973).

Black respondents report seeing their kin regularly either on a weekly or daily basis. In the McAdoo (1978) and Martineau (1977) studies, 20% and 40% respectively, of the respondents indicated seeing their relatives on a daily basis. Weekly visits seem to be the norm, with the majority of respondents reporting interaction of that frequency (Martineau, 1977). This pattern of frequent interaction with kin seems to be a more salient feature for Black families than white families (Hays and Mindel, 1973). In spite of frequent interaction, Black families evaluate their contacts with kin as appropriate, rather than "too much." In one study 68% of respondents felt that the amount of contact with kin was right, while 28% wanted to have even more. Only 5% of the respondents in the particular sample indicated they felt overwhelmed by seeing their kin so often (McAdoo, 1981).

While Black families form social ties with and rely on kin more than friends or neighbors, their social systems include members of these two other groups. The actual composition of Black families' social systems may be broader than originally thought. For instance, Lein and Stueve (1979) report that women form social relationships and exchange systems primarily with other women, usually their immediate kin. Stack (1974) and McAdoo (1978, 1979) substantiate this finding for Black women. While social networks composed of women who are immediate kin (mothers and sisters) are the predominant participation style, one study indicates that social systems may consist of a wider range of persons. The system of immediate kin may be augmented by extended female kin (aunts, sisters, and mothers-in-law). In addition to immediate and extended kin, friends including co-workers and fictive kin (i.e., ''play cousins'') may also be included in Black families' networks (Malson, 1980).

b. Co-workers. Co-worker-friends are potential sources of intimates for women with strong labor force histories. They often can be relied on for support and mutual exchanges needed. Malson (1980) found that men as well as women co-workers were named as part of the support systems of Black working women. Co-workers were most often included in the social systems of women who had professional or clerical jobs and who had worked in the same occupation and location over a period of time.

c. Fictive kin. The absorption of non-kin into the existing familial structure has long been an attribute of Black life. While living within a household is one way of being absorbed into a family, in some cases persons not living with families are seen as part of them because they function in family-type roles. These persons are usually referred to as ''play sisters'' or ''cousins'' to communicate the closeness of the relationship. While this indicates the ability of Black families to adapt to support persons who are unrelated, it also indicates the purposeful development of social support where relationships are absent or where additional ones are needed. Like other studies, McAdoo (1981) found that 71% of the subjects in her study had relationships with fictive kin. They took the roles of sisters, brothers, aunts, and uncles. Seventy percent of her respondents also stated that they had relationships with fictive kin as they were growing up.

The role that men and older children often play within the categories identified above is seldom acknowledged or discussed. Two recent studies indicate that they make salient contributions to the system (Malson, 1980; Weiss, 1980). The majority of the families interviewed by Malson (1980) named males as members of their support systems. In most cases, they were relatives the women respondents felt close to and on whom they could rely for mutual aid. Married and formerly married women named men as helpful with child care tasks. Sometimes present and former husbands took care of children, provided transportation to and from child care arrangements, or could be relied on to pay for child care exchanges where money was involved. Women also felt that they could rely on boy friends, younger nephews or brothers for help when they needed it.

If families have adolescent children, these children often contribute to the household economy in the form of help with child care or domestic tasks. Often they care for children at odd times to bridge the gap between formal and family-based child care: before school, to and from bus stops or transportation, and after school (Malson, 1979). Equally important, they help run the household by performing tasks that mothers would have to do themselves or which might be done by hired help in families with higher incomes (Weiss, 1980).

2. Assumptions Underlying System Participation

The participation of Black families in mutual-aid systems has been attributed to many factors. One hypothesis is that mutual caring and willingness to provide aid are based on culturally inculcated values. Doing for others is part of an Afro-American tradition and passed on from generation to generation (Nobles, 1978). A second hypothesis explaining this phenomenon is the need for economic support. Particularly among the poor, there is a need to share food and services for family survival. Yet a third reason is the functional nature of these support systems and the services they provide. By participating in these mutual exchange systems, families receive help with childrearing and child care, or help when in stress, or have the choice of receiving services that they would otherwise receive from professionals (McAdoo, 1977).

People belong to and participate in support networks because of the implicit understandings that exist between persons who participate in an exchange. These understandings are referred to as reciprocity (Stack, 1974) or kin insurance (McAdoo, 1979). Concepts of cooperation and exchange are based on the belief that what is given will be returned or reciprocated in time. In Carol Stack's analysis of welfare-dependent families, assumptions of reciprocity were expressed by the proverb "what goes around, comes around," meaning what you do for me today, you may need at another time. Others may participate in mutual help exchanges because they believe in "kin insurance," that the persons they provide for today may be the ones to rely on in times of future trouble (McAdoo, 1979).

Relationships also develop because of feelings of responsibility to children who are viewed as a new and future generation. In these instances, members of the social system may be bound by feelings of obligation for the well-being of those who are young and dependent. Studies report that support networks are often formed to provide support for domestic tasks, child care, and childrearing (Stack, 1974). Child care support is usually cited as one of the primary functions provided by kin and friends (Hays and Mindel, 1973).

Malson (1980, 1981) found that mutual exchanges were often based on feelings about responsibility to young children. These feelings seemed to persist in spite of severed parental relationships. The importance of caring for children as a basis for maintaining social relationships was indicated by the continued involvement of fathers with children whether or not they were married to their children's mothers. Fathers' relatives also had a role in the lives of children even after marriages had dissolved, and in some cases where they were never formalized. Support of children is probably an issue that kin, in spite of past experiences, can rally around. Children represent the next generation on whom one can place the hopes for mobility and success not experienced by parents.

Overall participation in support systems is predicated on social ties based on personal relationships and mutual trust. One indication of the trust underlying such support systems is that often no explicit rules or parameters govern exchanges. Persons participating often do not know whether they will receive the same services they give, whether the services will be of the same quality, or when in the future they might be called on again to perform a favor. Such feelings of trust often develop over time with sustained periods of contact that are usually a part of family relationships.

3. The Functions of Support Systems

While support systems may develop as part of a cultural pattern due to economic necessity or a combination of cultural and economic factors, they can also develop because of the services they provide. In this case the support system is functional, providing assistance with things that immediate family members are unable to supply. They may also act as an alternative to institutions or professional services that the family may view as non-supportive and unresponsive to their particular needs, or as overseers in situations where a family wishes to maintain control or promote their own cultural values. Help with child care and childrearing, economic assistance, and emotional support are often cited as the functions support systems can provide (Hays and Mindel, 1973).

a. Child care and childrearing. One of the major functions of support systems among Black families is to supply assistance with child care and childrearing. This specialized function has been documented in most studies of Black families and informal systems of mutual aid (Hill, 1977; Stack, 1974; Hays and Mindel, 1973; McAdoo, 1978, Malson, 1980). Child care and childrearing support may range from care for a few hours after school or evenings to informally adopting children into households, as described by Hill in *Informal Adoption Among Families* (1977) and Stack in *All Our Kin* (1974). Those who supply help with children are usually immediate kin (mothers, siblings, older children), but often include extended kin (aunts, mothers-in-law, and sisters-in-law). These persons provide child care, help with childrearing tasks, help with children in stressful situations, and offer socialization advice and information. The formation of a network around this specific need promotes the sharing of information and services usually unavailable to more isolated nuclear families (Malson, 1981).

b. Economic assistance. The economic assistance that network members provide may be in one of three forms: monetary, in-kind services or exchanges, or domestic living arrangements. Family members and close friends may lend others small sums of money, help with regular bills, or pool resources to provide larger amounts for mortgage or college tuition payments if needed. They may also assist by giving haircuts, repairing small things around the house, helping with car repairs, or helping others to move. In addition, sharing quarters or living in close proximity to family members is economically advantageous in that it helps to reallocate economic resources and facilitates opportunities for exchanges.

Provision of economic support per se does not appear to be highly correlated with income (McAdoo, 1978). In some instances, it is given to bolster a family's meager resources. For instance, Stack (1973) reported that the four-generational cluster of kin of Viola Jackson shared monetary income from her husband's seasonal work, welfare payments, and the part-time earnings of teenage children. On the other hand, economic assistance may be given to boost the buying power or standard of living in two-earner families (McAdoo, 1979). In one study, 27% of the middle-class families interviewed had received financial help through their social support systems. This was usually to tide them through periods of unemployment or to help pull together large amounts of money, such as a down payment for a house.

  c. Psychological well-being. How social-support systems mediate stress and contribute to the well-being of members is one of the least studied aspects of support-system functioning. In general, support systems seem to act as buffers between the family and external forces. In Black families they may help to alleviate some of the pressures brought on by racism, economic inequality, and feelings of isolation and separateness brought about through exclusion and non-acceptance. Other problems that network members may help with include those pertaining to children, economic pressures, personal relationships, and dislocation due to mobility and geographic change.

  The most important function of social-support systems may be to provide someone to rely on, to listen and offer advice about problems and concerns. McAdoo (1977) hypothesizes that Black families turn to network members in lieu of professional therapy when families face problems or crises. Persons feel close to support network members and go to them when they face issues that they cannot solve alone or that are interfering with everyday functioning.

EMPIRICAL RESEARCH ON BLACK FAMILIES' SOCIAL-SUPPORT SYSTEMS

  Empirical studies of the support systems of Black families have concentrated on defining the characteristics of support systems among various Black family types and forms. While this research has not been extensive, enough work has been done on Black families of varying types that some general assessments of the nature of their particular systems can be made. As suggested by Allen (1978), this literature can be grouped into studies focusing on

Black families at different life-cycle stages, those with different structures, and those of different social classes.

1. Life-Cycle Stage

Although we can readily identify the life-cycle stages of families who are subjects in studies, research on this topic has not concentrated on Black family support systems as a life-cycle issue. Studies comparing the support systems of Black families at different life-cycle stages have yet to be conducted. Information about Blacks at particular stages of the family life cycle tends to be grouped at either end of the life-cycle continuum. Some studies focus on the support systems of families with young children, particularly those who are preschoolers and elementary school aged (Stack, 1974; McAdoo, 1978, 1979, 1980). Others examine support systems in later life-cycle stages, particularly the empty-nest phase, when elderly women have no dependent children of their own to care for (Hill, 1977; Jackson, 1978). There is little work exploring the characteristics of the support systems of Black families at the life-cycle stages falling between. For instance, the literature offers little concerning the support systems of families who have adolescents and teenagers, a stage where psychological support for parenting is often needed.

The bulk of the literature on Black families' social systems concentrates on families with young children. Presumably, support and mutual aid are needed more at this time than other times within a family's span. More importantly, this literature hypothesizes that Black family support systems are often based on relationships and mutual-aid systems that provide for the well-being of young children. Help with childrearing is a typical form of aid supplied by support system members and is cited as one of the main ways in which families may supply help to each other (Hays and Mindel, 1973). Stack (1974) felt that much of the support exchanged in the kin systems she observed was organized around child care and childrearing support. Likewise, McAdoo (1979) found that child care help was the most prevalent type of help that single parent families said that they received from network members. The importance of childrearing help as a supportive resource to Black families is exemplified in a study by Malson (1981) identifying specialized subsystems of childrearing support that Black families rely on for child care and childrearing aid.

In addition to studies of the early life cycle phases of Black families, there are also those looking at support systems in later family life-cycle phases. The support systems of Black families with elderly women as heads is a frequent topic. Hill's study of informal adoption in Black families dispelled some myths and stereotypes about this particular extended family form. One widely held stereotype is that the typical Black extended family consists of a young nuclear family with an elderly woman, usually a mother of the husband or wife, living with them. The opposite living situation is in fact more likely to be in case. Elderly women are more likely to incorporate young families or dependent children into their own households. Hill (1977) points out that only 4% of Black families had elderly persons 65 years of age or older living with them.

Black families headed by elderly women provide mutual aid and assistance to other family members primarily through shared living arrangements. Dependent children, usually grandchildren, or subfamilies consisting of females and young children, are absorbed into the primary family unit. In 1974, half of the Black families with elderly female heads had children under 18 years of age who were not their own living with them. (Hill and Shakleford, 1978).

Families headed by elderly Black women contribute substantially to support and mutual-aid systems in spite of meager resources to share. They tend to have some of the lowest incomes in the United States. In 1969, when Robert Hill gathered his data, the median income of these families with informally adopted children was $1,632. In contrast, two-parent Black families with informally adopted children had a median income of $3,769; one-parent Black families with informally adopted children had a median income of $2,500.

Jackson (1978) examined the social relationships and the mutual-aid systems of grandmothers and grandfathers in urban areas in the South. She was particularly interested in explaining whether characteristics of the support and mutual-aid systems (such as informal adoption) were shared by grandparents of different ages, with different living arrangements, and by grandfathers as well as grandmothers. Kin relationships in these families were similar to those in studies of white families and not indicative of powerful matriarchies.

Grandmothers who had daughters interacted more frequently with their grandchildren than those who had sons who were parents. Younger grandparents in this study were more likely to share residences with grandchildren than were older ones. The majority of the grandparents had received assistance from their grandchildren in the preceding year. The form of aid varied, with those grandparents who lived alone receiving more visits from grandchildren than those grandparents living with other family members, and those grandparents living with other family members receiving more help with household or yard work than grandparents living alone. In turn, most grandparents, regardless of living arrangements, helped with child care.

Most grandparents interviewed in this study said that they preferred their grandchildren living near them and not with them. While this finding seems to contradict findings from the Hill (1977) study about the number of grandparents caring for dependent children, it may foretell changes in informal adoption patterns accompanying migration from rural to urban settings. Since informal adoption of children by elderly families headed by women is primarily a southern rural phenomenon, Black grandparents may exhibit similar living preferences as they become more urban and are in northern rather than southern locations.

2a. Two-Parent Families

Studies of the support systems of Black families with young children have included either two-parent or single-parent families, or both (Hays and Mindell, 1973; McAdoo, 1978, 1979, 1980, 1981). One might say that two-parent families have been subjects in studies of Black families' social networks. In reality, these studies have been interested in other hypotheses, e.g., mobility, and not the characteristics of the support systems of two-parent families, or the role of these systems in the functioning of these families. Based on such studies we do know that two-parent families informally absorb children in their households (Hill, 1977); that two-parent Black elderly families participate in Black families mutual-aid systems (Jackson, 1978); and that two-parent families participate in child care exchanges as a model form of mutual aid (Hays and Mindel, 1973; McAdoo, 1978).

Two-parent families in which both parents are employed are one variation of this family form. One of the gaps in the empirical research on Black families and social networks is the absence of information about the role of mutual-aid systems in dual-earner

Black families. With a background of work and career that has
been judged as both a family asset and liability, there have been
many projections about why Black women have been able to work
outside the home and maintain their families while other women,
prior to the "subtle revolution" (Smith, 1979) have not. One hypothesis about this ability is that the mutual-aid systems among
Black families has provided child care and domestic support for
Black families in which mothers are employed (McAdoo, 1978).
Although this is a rather widely held assumption, no study has
stated as its purpose describing or deciphering the role of support
systems in buffering the stress accompanying role overload in
Black work or dual career families.

2b. One-Parent Families

More work has been done on the support systems of Black
single parent families. The works of Stack (1974), Malson (1980,
1981), and McAdoo (1981) provide information on the life of
Black women who head families. This work indicates that support
network members provide aid not only in times of crisis but in an
ongoing fashion, easing stressful situations. It supports the hypothesis that Black families have adjusted to the demands of the single-
parent role because of help received from support system members.

In most instances, parenting alone does not precisely describe
the situations of Black women who are single and bringing up children. Family members seem to be aware of what single parenting
demands from adults and seem predisposed to making contributions. While one-way exchanges are not expected, participation
in systems where "favors" are given and received seems to be a
common occurrence. For instance, 61% of the single parents in
one study reported receiving a great deal of help from kin
(McAdoo, 1979).

Living arrangements used as part of the mutual-aid system have
been particularly beneficial to Black single-parent families. While
sub-families are only 6% of all Black families, they are over-
whelmingly attenuated, consisting of females and their young children (Hill and Shakleford, 1978). Most live in the homes of relatives, usually their parents, or in some cases, their sisters. Often
this is done so that the mother can work or to provide more economic security to the family through "doubling up" and sharing

resources. Also, shared living arrangements can provide support to very young or teenage mothers whom the family may view as too immature to be solely responsible for childrearing (Hill and Shakleford, 1978).

A pilot study of the support strategies of Black single parent families investigated how these systems helped women parenting alone cope with their roles of breadwinner and homemaker/child-rearer (Malson, 1980). Ten Black women parenting alone were interviewed as part of Favors: The Support Systems of Urban Black Women and Their Families, conducted in collaboration with Dr. Laura Lein. All had preschool or elementary school aged children and were primarily responsible for domestic tasks. The majority worked or attended school. Some seemed to function extremely well in spite of their multiple responsibilities. For instance, one woman who had older children was a peer group counselor for other single parents; three women were attending college and one single parent who began work 15 years ago as a domestic now owned her own business.

All identified a support network that ranged in size from 30 to 104 persons, and averaged 63 members. The range of persons who might supply help seemed to have more variation than that reported in other studies of women's social networks (Lein and Stueve, 1979; Stack, 1974; McAdoo, 1978, 1979). Besides immediate kin (mothers and sisters), women also named extended kin (aunts, sisters, mothers-in-law, and quasi-kin); friends, including co-workers; men; and older children. Support network members helped with financial support, child care and domestic tasks, and emotional well-being through willingness to discuss topics about which single women were concerned.

These women did not appear to have conflict about the duality of their commitments nor to be overly concerned about accomplishing them well. The majority seemed to have adapted to single-parenting life. Most wished that they had more time in which to do what they had to do, but said that they felt overwhelmed only once in a while. They also reported that they were pretty happy, often felt proud or pleased with themselves, and felt things would turn out well for them.

Harriette McAdoo is currently investigating Black single-parent families and how they cope with the stress associated with work and childrearing. These mothers are active support-system members, and some (15%) wish they could have closer contact with their families. Emotional support, financial help, child care, and children's clothing are exchanged among members. Child care seems to be the most frequently exchanged item. Mothers have indicated that while they prefer having children taken care of by relatives or close friends, they use day care centers because most friends and family members work.

The amount of stress faced by these mothers varies. Some have very low levels of stress (as measured by the Holmes and Roche Scale) and report experiencing few stressful life events in the past two years. One significant finding is that stress levels differ by marital status and income with levels being higher for mothers who had been married previously, with incomes above the median, and middle and lower class mothers. When asked to identify the sources that caused the most stress, mothers mention income, housing, and work. Little stress is associated with parenting concerns or personal relationships.

In summary, while support-network resources have recently been recognized as a source contributing to family functioning, the Black extended family has always been recognized as a source of emotional strength and mutual aid (Hill, 1971). Within this system, Black women and Black men extend support to Black women parenting alone. Members of social-support systems have been instrumental in promoting and contributing to the survival and maintenance of Black single parents. This extended support system functions to supplement the tasks that a parent may be unable to accomplish, to counteract strains that a family might experience, and to help stabilize what has been seen as an unorganized family pattern.

3. Social Class

Hypotheses about support systems among Black families of different social classes have been based on two competing notions. The first is that support and mutual-aid systems are established primarily because of economic need. Support systems are survival mechanisms which are present at times when families are most vulnerable. For instance, Stack's work indicates that mutual-aid systems are primarily established to redistribute sparse economic resources among families in poverty. The second notion is that these support systems exist regardless of economic need and are present because they are an Afro-American cultural pattern (Nobles, 1978; McAdoo, 1978, 1979). Therefore, support systems and evidence of mutual aid will be an aspect of Black family life regardless of social class.

These two hypotheses imply different conceptions of the assumptions underlying social-support systems. The economic thesis implies that participants have to be in a certain state of need to respect the reciprocal obligations that make the system function. If this need is not present, or if more affluent families have the option of purchasing goods and services they might otherwise barter, the reciprocal social bonds that the system is based on might diminish and the system itself fall apart in the process.

The cultural thesis implies that persons participate in mutual aid systems because it is consonant with their belief and value system to look out for one another. Middle class families, then, share resources not motivated by the value of what they get back but because they probably have been helped in the past and might need help in the future. For even when higher economic status is established, Black middle class families need help from others to achieve income parity with middle class families who are white (McAdoo, 1978).

Against the framework of economic and cultural hypotheses, researchers have looked at the support systems of working class and middle class families. Hays and Mindel (1973) interviewed Black families primarily of lower class status in one of the only studies investigating kinship support among Black and white families in the same social class. Besides socioeconomic status, this study also controlled for number of relatives and geographic mobility of 25 matched pairs of families. The investigators found that Black families saw more kin (except parents) and saw them more often than their white counterparts. In addition, using child care as a prototype service, Black families were found to receive more help and receive it more often than white families. These families were more likely to have kin living with them (28% as compared to 4% of the white families), but they were siblings or children and not parents. Kin were also perceived as more salient people in the lives of families who were Black.

Hays and Mindel (1973) interpreted their findings as evidence of the more prevalent existence among Blacks of families that extended beyond nuclear family boundaries. These families were centered less around parent-child relationships, as evidenced by the range of kin other than parents that subjects interacted with. The investigators also hypothesized that the solidarity of sibling ties and the absorption of children into families was an indication of less dependence by Blacks on nuclear family models.

Harriette MacAdoo (1978) investigated the support systems in middle class families to substantiate their presence in families who were economically stable and to explore their role in fostering and maintaining mobility. With a sample of 174 mothers and 131 fathers representing 178 family units, she found that kin exchange systems were "alive and well" among the middle class. Most respondents (85%) had moved into as opposed to being born in (15%) the middle class. Financial, emotional, and child care help were exchanged as part of the system. Respondents indicated that they received the same level of help from kin before and after mobility. Those participating in the support systems of families who were newly mobile had the highest expectations for sharing resources. Evidence from this study supports the hypothesis that systems of mutual aid among Black families are not motivated solely by economic need.

In summary, work showing evidence of social-support systems among Black families of different types supports the hypotheses that self-help systems, especially among kin, are characteristic of them (Nobles, 1978). Research on families in different structures and with different social class backgrounds shows support systems which are similarly organized and with similar functions. Additional studies might investigate family types which have not been examined or conduct comparative analyses of support systems among Black families in different life-cycle phases.

CONCLUDING REMARKS

The study of the support systems of Black families, like the study of Black families in general, is in its early stages. While our knowledge of this topic has grown, particularly in the last decade, researchers on Black families should be aware of the existing gaps in our knowledge and the need to advance our understanding of the role support systems play in faciliating Black family functional adaptation.

Approaches and methodologies used to study this topic have been diverse. The new national surveys on Black Americans will add to our understanding of social relations and social support among Black families. In addition to large scale surveys that are representative and generalizable to all Black Americans, we also need small intensive studies that focus on specific aspects of these systems or which compare systems among different kinds of Black families. For instance, the assumptions underlying mutual-aid systems among Black families should be investigated. Work on the support systems of Black families in different life-cycle stages must be conducted to advance Black family theory in general. The role of support systems in facilitating adaptive family functioning in single-parent and dual-career families might be the prototype for studying adaptation mechanisms. A study on this topic might indicate how and if support systems function as the margin of error, the strategic variable that facilitates adaptive functioning and in some cases family survival.

New studies should explore both the advantages and disadvantages to system participation (Belle, 1981). The persons close to and relied on by an individual are often themselves the source of stress. Sometimes this is a drawback of personal-social relationships. The benefits and the costs, not necessarily expressed in monetary terms, of involvement in social-support systems for Black families should be examined.

Knowledge of Black family social-support systems might have positive and negative consequences for policy formation and the establishment of social programs. There may be a tendency, by some, to conclude that social programs are not necessary because Black families seem to be helping each other adequately enough. The existence of informal child care arrangements has fostered this perspective among opponents of federally sponsored day care programs (Woolsey, 1977). Therefore, studies of the relationship between these systems among Black families, policy analysis, and program design should be encouraged.

NOTES

1. This paper will not, for example, include early works on Black social-support systems and the extended family such as the work of E. Franklin Frazier (1939) *The Negro Family in the United States.*

2. Two recent surveys begun in the late seventies will greatly increase our knowledge of the prevalence of Black families' social-support systems by providing empirical data based on national surveys of Black Americans. The first, the National Survey of Black Americans (NSBA) directed by James Jackson at the Institute for Survey Research, University of Michigan, is based on data collected from a national probability sample of 2,000 Black Americans. Included in the questionnaire of over 1,000 items are many questions about so-

cial support and help-seeking. The second, the National Black Pulse Survey, conducted by the National Urban League, also has a strong emphasis on the support systems of Black families.

3. While I have dichotomized the empirical research in this area into work that has economic or cultural theoretical orientations, Black family researchers recognize that these variables often interact to influence the presence and patterns of social-support systems.

REFERENCES

Allen, W. R. Black family research in the United States: A review, assessment and extension. *Journal of Comparative Family Studies,* 1978, *9,* 167–190.

Allen, W. R. Class, culture, and family organization: The effects of class and race on family structure in urban America. *Journal of Comparative Family Studies,* 1979, *10,* 301–314.

Aschenbrenner, J. Extended families among Black Americans. *Journal of Comparative Studies,* 1973, *4,* 257-268.

Aschenbrenner, J. *Lifelines: Black families in Chicago.* New York: Holt, Rinehart and Winston, 1975.

Belle, D. The social network as a source of both stress and support to low-income mothers. Paper presented at the meeting of the Society for Research in Child Development, Boston, April 1981.

Billingsley, A. *Black families in White America.* Englewood Cliffs, NJ: Prentice Hall, Inc., 1968.

Billingsley, A., and J. Giovannoni. *Children of the storm.* New York: Harcourt, Brace Jovanovich, 1972.

Frazier, E. F. *The Negro family in the United States.* Chicago, IL: University of Chicago Press, 1939.

Gutman, H. *The Black family in slavery and freedom.* New York: Vintage, 1976.

Hays, W. C., and Mindel, C. H. Extended kinship relations in black and white families. *Journal of Marriage and the Family,* 1973, *35,* 51–56.

Hill, R. *The strengths of Black families.* New York: Emerson Hall, 1972.

Hill, R. *Informal adoption among Black families.* Washington, DC: National Urban League, 1977.

Hill, R., and Shakleford, L. The Black extended family revisited. In Robert Staples (Ed.), *The Black family: Essays and studies.* Belmont, CA: Wadsworth Publishing Co., 1978, 201–206.

Jackson, J. Black grandparents in the South. In R. Staples (Ed.), *The Black family.* Belmont, CA: Wadsworth Co., 1978.

McAdoo, H. Family therapy in the Black community. *American Journal of Orthopsychiatry,* 1977, *47.*

McAdoo, H. Factors related to stability in upwardly mobile Black families. *Journal of Marriage and the Family,* 1978, *40,* 761–776.

McAdoo, H. Black kinship. *Psychology Today,* May 1979.

McAdoo, H. Black mothers and the extended family support network. In La Frances Rodgers-Rose, (Ed.), *The Black women.* Beverly Hills, CA: Sage Publications, Inc., 1980.

McAdoo, H. Stress and support networks of working single Black mothers. Paper delivered at the meeting of the Society for Research on Child Development, Boston, April 1981.

Malson, M. Child care decision making: Families, childrearing support networks and social policy. Unpublished doctoral dissertation, Harvard University, 1979.

Malson, M. Favors: A pilot study of the support systems of urban Black women and their families. Unpublished paper, Wellesley College Center for Research on Women, 1980.

Malson, M. Black families and childrearing support networks. Paper delivered at the meeting of the Society for Research on Child Development, Boston, April 1981.

Malson, M. Black women, work and family life. Work in progress, Wellesley College Center for Research on Women.

Martin, E., Martin, J. M. *The Black extended family*. Chicago: The University of Chicago Press, 1978.

Martineau, W. Informal social ties among urban Black Americans. *Journal of Black Studies*, 1977, *9*, 83–104.

Nobles, W. Toward an empirical and theoretical framework for defining Black families. *Journal of Marriage and the Family*, 1978, *40*, 679–688.

Pleck, E. *Black migration and poverty*. New York: Academic Press, 1980.

Smith, R. E. (Ed.) *The subtle revolution*. Washington, DC: The Urban Institute, 1979.

Stack, C. The kindred of Viola Jackson. In N. E. Whitten and J. Szeved (Eds.), *Afro-American anthropology: Contemporary perspectives*. New York: The Free Press, 1973.

Stack, C. *All our kin*. New York: Harper, 1974.

Taylor, R. J. The informal social support networks of Black Americans: A preliminary analysis from the National Survey of Black Americans. Paper presented at the Thirteenth Annual Conference of the National Association of Black Social Workers, April 1981.

U.S. Department of Labor. *Monthly Labor Review*, 1979, *120*, 39.

Walker, K. N., MacBride, A., and Vachon, M. L. S. Social support networks and the crisis of bereavement. *Social Science and Medicine*, 1977, *11*, 35–41.

Weiss, R. S. Growing up a little faster: The experience of growing up in a single-parent household. *Journal of Social Issues*. 1979, *35*, 97–111.

Woolsey, S. H. Pied piper politics and the child-care debate. *Daedalus*, 1977, *106*, 127.

Working Family Project. Work and Family Life. Final Report to the National Institutes of Education, 1974.

The Elderly as Network Members

Ann Stueve

Despite efforts to alter our images of old age as a particularly needy or dependent stage of life, research on social networks and the elderly all too often focuses on older men and women as recipients of support and as reliant upon the caregiving efforts of others. This focus reflects a concern with how the elderly experience and deal with some of the difficult and often stressful events and conditions associated with old age—widowhood, the death of friends, retirement, frailty, and the accumulation of chronic illnesses and disabilities. Since the purpose of much of this research is to further our understanding of how people use their social networks to adapt to both the routine and unexpected demands of growing older and to inform policy-makers about the kinds of strategies which are most effective in creating and bolstering support systems, this approach is both necessary and justifiable. However, by calling attention to older people as recipients of services, it tends to overstate the extent to which the elderly are passive beneficiaries of the labors of others and act as a drain on the energy and resources of those closest to them. More importantly, it tends to understate the extent to which older men and women contribute to their social networks by providing services, engaging in reciprocal exchanges, and helping others, both old and young, cope with the stressful events in their own lives.

This paper draws from the literature on aging and social networks in order to examine the active role older people play both as members of the informal networks of their families, friends, and neighbors and as participants in more formal settings within the wider community. Looking at the elderly from this vantage point is important not only because many obtain support through their interactions with older people but also because the elderly them-

Ann Stueve is in the Graduate Program in Sociology, University of California at Berkeley.

selves derive a sense of usefulness and well-being from what they give as well as receive. Moreover, in providing help to others, older people increase the likelihood that they will receive support as well. As Wentowski (1979) notes, "certain implicit rules of reciprocity govern people's exchanges of support" (p. 8). By extending aid to others, the elderly people she observed signaled their willingness to engage in a relationship of mutual give and take; by accepting help, they tacitly acknowledged their willingness eventually to repay.

A characterization of the elderly as active network contributors and community participants is out of step with many of our cultural images and beliefs about old age. While stereotypes of senile or debilitated old people are not widely held (Lutsky, 1980), nevertheless, the image of old age as a period of inactivity and passivity persists. Results from the Louis Harris and Associates' (1975) survey, for example, indicate that most respondents between the ages of 18 and 64 saw "most people over 65" as spending "a lot of time" watching television (68%) and sitting and thinking (66%); additionally, substantial minorities believed that most older people spend a lot of time gardening or raising plants (47%), reading (45%), sleeping (42%), and just doing nothing (37%). In every case these percentages exceeded the proportion of elderly respondents (65 years or older) who reported devoting considerable time to such sedentary—and for the most part solitary—activities. Moreover, while older interviewees were less likely to ascribe such an inactive and unsociable life-style to "most people over 65," in several cases, many of the elderly, too, tended to view their contemporaries as engaging in relatively passive activities (even though they themselves did not report doing so).

Dependency and the loss of self-reliance are additional images associated with old age. Two of the more common refrains in interviews with older people are their stated desires to remain independent and to avoid becoming a "burden on my children." Many adult children also express concerns and anxieties about what the future may hold, even when elderly parents are still viewed as active and functioning adults (e.g., Cicirelli, 1981; Neugarten, 1979). In recent years we have witnessed the airing of many documentaries and news specials focusing on such questions as "what should be done about mom and dad?" (WCVB, 1981) as well as the proliferation of advice books written for children with aging parents. While such media events and publications respond to a real need on the part of many families for information and help in dealing with the psychological and service needs of old family members, they can also capitalize on the fears of young and old and fuel the image of old age as a period of dependency and a cause of family problems, especially when they are marketed with such titles as *Survival Handbook for Children of Aging Parents* (Schwartz, 1977) and *The Other Generation Gap* (Cohen and Gans, 1978).

Focusing on the elderly as active contributors to their families and communities also deviates from that stream of gerontological thought which emphasizes the problematic side of old age. Concepts such as parent-caring, role reversal, and filial crisis carry the implication that mothers and fathers become psychologically and materially dependent as they grow old and that this dependency, in turn, poses problems for their families. Similarly, current assessments of the state of the modern family also tend to characterize the aging of parents as problematic. For example, many have speculated that the increased labor force participation of adult daughters will limit the amount of care families are able and willing to provide and increase the stresses entailed in meeting the needs of the old (e.g., Brody, 1979; Pilisuk and Minkler, 1980; Shanas, 1980; Treas, 1977).

Both the pervasiveness and inaccuracy of such images are reflected in the unwillingness of substantial proportions of people over 65 to label themselves as elderly (see Turner, 1979, for a review) and the reluctance of many of their close associates to identify them as old as well. "Being old" is associated with poor health and needing help from others (Bultena and Powers, 1978), not self-reliance or the giving of support; these are the province of young adulthood and especially middle-age. Hence, many chronologically old people continue to identify with the middle-aged because they remain socially active and capable adults. While there is no denying that when older people are in difficulty they generally turn to family members, especially daughters, for help (Cicirelli, 1981; Lopata, 1979; Shanas, 1979) and that prolonged or intensive caregiving is a difficult enterprise for families to take on and manage alone (e.g., Archbold, 1978; Isaacs et al., 1972), it should also be emphasized that the image of elderly people as inactive, passive, and dependent is only accurate for a segment of the population and only for a portion of that life stage we call old age.

First, for most, old age is not a brief span of time but a prolonged period of years. In 1975, for example, people who reached their 65th birthday could on the average expect to live another 16 years (Kovar, 1977). Second, even though many experience spells of illness or adapt to living with some chronic diseases, the majority remain in good health. Interviews with older people conducted by the National Center for Health Statistics (ibid.) found that 69% rated their health as excellent or good; only 9% rated their health as poor. In a similar survey in Massachusetts, 50% of the people interviewed who were 85 years and older said they were in excellent or good health while only 17% rated their health as poor (Branch, 1977). Third, recent figures also indicate that only about 4% to 6% of the population 65 years and older (and approximately one-fifth of those 80 years and older) suffer from organic brain syndrome (Raskind and Storric, 1980), and medical advances are beginning to help some of those who do experience disease-related mental deterioration in old age. Finally, growing old does not always entail a progressive accumulation of mental, physical, and social losses leading to ever-increasing needs for support. Older people do recover from illnesses and fractures, adapt to disabilities, remarry or adjust to widowhood, and the like. For the most part, it is the very old who are most limited in their daily activities and most in need of day-to-day help.

Given that most older people are in relatively good health for much of the time, it is not surprising that they remain engaged in social relationships which entail giving help and support as well as receiving it. Although there is evidence (much cross-sectional) suggesting that the average size of social networks decreases with old age (e.g., Stueve and Fischer, 1978; see Lowenthal and Robinson, 1976, for a review) and that older individuals tend to exhibit increased interiority (Cohler and Lieberman, 1979; Neugarten, 1973; Neugarten et al., 1964), most elderly maintain involvement in social exchanges, particularly with those who are closest to them. As with all age groups, there is much variation in the types and extent of contacts which are sustained, ranging from the relatively marginal ties of residents of inner city hotels to the close-knit family ties of certain ethnic groups to the often supportive friendship bonds which can develop in retirement communities. In the following, I review what is known about the elderly as contributors to their networks, moving from a discussion of the elderly as family members, to looking at the elderly as friends and neighbors, and concluding with an examination of the role the elderly play in their communities.

THE ELDERLY AS FAMILY MEMBERS

While our images of extended families in past generations include elderly aunts and uncles, grandparents and great-grandparents, it is only with recent increases in life expectancy and the survival of most people to age 65 and beyond that older relatives have become commonplace in the majority of families. As Brody (1979) points out, "in contrast to earlier periods of history, when most marriages were broken by death by the time the last child left home, many people now reach adulthood during the lifetimes of their grandparents, and many more children have great-grandparents" (p. 270). One ramification of this shift is a wider variety of potential family relationships for older people. Surveys indicate that approximately four-fifths of the population 65 and older who have ever married have living children (Troll et al., 1979); approximately three-quarters of those who have had children are grandparents (ibid.), and two-fifths or more are great-grandparents (Neugarten, 1979; Shanas, 1980). Black elderly, in particular, are likely to head four-generation families, with about 47% doing so (Lipman, personal communication).

Along with ties to younger generations, a small (but probably growing) proportion of elderly still have parents alive. Among respondents to the Harris and Associates' (1975) survey, 4% reported at least one living parent. Looking at it from the reverse direction, Troll et al. (1979) estimate that approximately 10% of the population 65 years and older have children who are 65 or older as well. There is little information on the numbers of elderly with living aunts, uncles, or parents-in-law, but clearly, for a segment of the elderly population, family relations extend upward as well as downward.

In addition to these vertical, or intergenerational, relations, horizontal family ties are also common. Approximately seven out of ten people 75 years and older reported at least one living sibling in 1975 (Shanas, 1979). Marital relationships are prevalent for older men, though not for older women. Given the greater longevity of women and their tendency to select husbands who are a few years older, elderly women are much more likely to be widowed and living alone. In 1978, for example, less than half (46%) of all women

65 to 74 years were married and living with a spouse compared to nearly four-fifths (78%) of all similarly aged men; the disparity was even more pronounced among those 75 years and older, with only 22% of all women married compared to 68% of all men (Soldo, 1980). Elderly widowers are also more likely to remarry than widows (Morgan, 1979).

The mere existence of family members, of course, does not guarantee that older people maintain active relationships with their kin. Although it has become virtually a tenet of faith that kinship ties persist in the United States and that the ''modified extended family'' is the predominant form, some researchers are beginning to question the extent to which continuous and extensive exchanges of social and material support actually characterize family relations. Lopata (1979), for example, argues that most research supporting the modified extended family thesis has focused almost exclusively on interactions between parents and adult children and not on exchanges with less immediate kin; moreover, much of the help that people report occurs around life course transitions or during periods of crisis. Based on a survey of young and old widows, she concludes that ''members of the kin network, such as parents, brothers, sisters, 'other relatives' meaning grandparents, aunts and uncles, cousins and grandchildren are generally unavailable and rarely appear in the support systems of the Chicago area widows represented by our sample'' (p. 231; see also Matthews, 1979, and Stueve and Fischer, 1978, for similar analyses).

In part, the issue of to what extent the modified extended family exists is one of degree and interpretation: How much interaction and support are necessary to label an older person as integrated into a web of kinship ties and associations? In contrast to Lopata, Shanas (1979), for example, emphasizes the involvement of old people in kinship networks, based on results from a 1975 survey of non-institutionalized people 65 years and older. Three-quarters of those interviewed who had offspring either lived in the same household as a child or within a thirty-minute drive; a similar proportion had seen a child within the past week. One-third of the respondents with living siblings had seen a brother or sister within the last seven days, and about three in ten interviewees had visited with some relative other than a child, grandchild, or sibling in this same time period. These data clearly demonstrate Shanas' contention that most older people are far from isolated from their kin. However, they also support Lopata's argument that frequent interaction is much more prevalent between elderly parents and their children than with the wider kin community. In addition, the results skim over the question of whether most older people have such regular interaction with all or most of their offspring (or sibs or other relatives) or with just one or two. Finally, as Shanas (1979, 1980) herself points out, such findings provide little information on the quality of kinship relations or on the extent to which visits are perfunctory rituals or occasions of mutual give and take.

With this introductory profile, the rest of this section examines the family relations of older people, beginning with ties to older generations, then turning to horizontal bonds, and concluding with ties to younger generations. In doing so, it focuses on the extent to which older people are involved in providing support as well as on the stresses and joys they experience as a result of their active participation in kinship exchanges.

Ties to Older Generations

One of the increasingly important ways that older people contribute to the lives of others is as children of elderly parents and parents-in-law. Yet, aside from census and survey data on living arrangements, general information on elderly parent/adult child ties and anecdotal accounts, little is known about the content or quality of the relation between very old parents (typically mothers) and their near-old or young-old children. Many have speculated that this relationship is likely to contain elements of parent-caring since very old people are more apt to be infirm and that caregiving is likely to be stressful since many children may be facing problems and difficulties associated with their own aging. The first conjecture is probably accurate; the second is more open to question.

Much research on the support systems of the elderly confirms the importance of children, especially daughters, in providing help and sustaining the elderly through periods of need (e.g., Cantor, 1979; Shanas, 1979, 1980). While few (if any) studies have explicitly addressed the situation of elderly children with elderly parents, it is likely that daughters in their 60s and early 70s respond in ways similar to their mid-life counterparts, providing social contacts and emotional support, helping with shopping and transportation, making themselves available in times of illness, and the like. To date, however, there has been little documentation of the extent to which elderly children provide support to the very old or the ways in which support is patterned within families. For example, are elderly children less likely to become involved in intensive caregiving if there are younger siblings available to provide support?

An additional question concerns how elderly men and women experience their role as children of very old parents, whether they find it rewarding and fulfilling or taxing and a strain. It is likely that elderly children who have health problems of their own find activities and responsibilities associated with parent-caring stressful, if not impossible. However, as indicated above, most people in their 60s and early 70s are in reasonable health, and how they experience the demands of parent-caring is unclear. Theories of role conflict might suggest that elderly children are in a better position to undertake parent-caring activities than younger adults, who are more apt to be enmeshed in a variety of competing employment, parenting, and community roles (see O'Donnell's review in this issue). Alternatively, parent-caring may be more of an intrusion during the "empty nest" and retirement years, which are often looked forward to because of the freedom they offer, than in earlier life stages when much of men's and women's lives are already constrained and shaped by the needs of others, especially children. Clearly, before labeling elderly children as particularly burdened or stressed, we need to know more about how elderly children aid and support relatives even older than themselves as well as about the joys and stresses involved in such relations.

Horizontal Ties to Spouses and Siblings

The marital relationship is the most obvious context in which many older men and women contribute to the well-being of others. As Troll et al. (1979) conclude from their review of research on older marriages, "for the happily married older couple, marriage is central to the 'good life.' It is a source of great comfort and support as well as the focal point of everyday life" (p. 53). While clearly not all elderly husbands and wives are happily married, nevertheless, several cross-sectional studies indicate that elderly couples tend to report greater satisfaction and contentment with their marriages than couples in the active child-rearing years (Feldman, 1964, cited in Troll et al., 1979; Orthner, 1975; Rollins and Cannon, 1974; Stinnett et al., 1972). There is also evidence to suggest that marriage insulates at least some groups of elderly from some of the problems and worries associated with growing older. Hutchison (1975), for example, found that married individuals whose incomes were low but above the poverty line were less likely to feel lonely, unhappy, worried, and dissatisfied with their lives than their unmarried counterparts, though marriage did not act as a strong enough buffer for elderly whose incomes left them in poverty. Being married (as well as having children) also appears to delay, if not always prevent, institutionalization in old age (Brody et al., 1978; Johnson, 1980; Vincente et al., 1979; Wan, 1980).

Although there have been few attempts to specify what it is about marriage that protects older people from stressful events or helps them cope with difficult situations that do arise, there are a number of ways in which older husbands and wives act as important bases of help and support. Wives, for example, tend to be primary sources of confidant relationships for older men, though elderly women themselves often look outside of marriage to female friends and relatives for intimate associations (Brown, 1980; Fischer and Phillips, 1979; Lowenthal and Haven, 1968; Powers and Bultena, 1976). Husbands, by virtue of their greater lifetime earnings and higher retirement incomes, provide their wives with more economic resources than are generally available to women who are widowed, divorced, or who never married (e.g., Miller, 1977; Thompson, 1977). Where relationships are good, husbands and wives provide one another with companionship and help with household work. Studies examining the division of household labor generally indicate considerable sharing of tasks on the part of elderly couples (Atchley and Miller, 1980; Kerckhoff, 1966), especially when contrasted with the sex-differentiated patterns typically reported by men and women in the midst of raising children (see O'Donnell's review in this issue).

In addition to these day-to-day forms of support, elderly husbands and wives play a particularly critical role as help-givers when spouses are ill or infirm. While much attention has been directed to the problems children experience in caring for elderly parents, it must be remembered that when both parents are alive, spouses—not children—tend to be the primary source of help and support (Cantor, 1977, 1980; Lewis et al., 1980; Shanas, 1979). This caregiving at times may be extensive and prolonged. In her first study of widowhood, Lopata (1973) found that nearly half

(46%) of the widows interviewed had kept their husbands at home during their final illnesses, and about two-fifths of these women had provided care for more than a year. While elderly wives are more likely to be thrust into a caregiving role because of their greater longevity, Shanas' (1977) research indicates that elderly husbands also take on caregiving responsibilities when wives are ill. As she puts it, "men take over traditionally female tasks as necessary, women find strength to turn and lift bedfast husbands" (quoted in Tobin and Kulys, 1980, p. 378).

Research by Johnson (1980) also suggests that spouses may be the more preferable caregivers. Locating a sample of 167 elderly patients who had recently been discharged from acute-care hospitals, she compared the experiences of those primarily cared for by a spouse (45%) with those tended by a child (35%). In general, husbands and wives tended to provide more comprehensive and continuous services, to feel less stressed, to report fewer competing commitments, and to accept the role of caregiver with fewer reservations. Elderly patients were more satisfied with the care provided by spouses, and less conflict was reported by all concerned.

Of course, caring for an ailing spouse is not without costs. Johnson (1980), for example, notes the relative isolation experienced by many of the elderly couples she interviewed. When spouses were available to provide support, other family members tended to withdraw and let the elderly couples manage on their own. Moreover, additional problems ensued when both partners were frail or in failing health. Others have also pointed to the social isolation, emotional strain, and sheer physical work that caregiving can entail, especially when the need for support is long-term (Crossman et al., 1981; Fengler and Goodrich, 1979).

Siblings. While there is little doubt that spouses play a central role in the support systems of older people, there is less consensus (and less research) on the extent to which siblings provide one another with help and support in old age. Lopata (1979) contends that brothers and sisters were quite inactive, both as providers and as recipients of aid, in the support systems of the widows she interviewed. Looking back, only half of the widows reported that their families of orientation were generally helpful during the time they were setting up new lives, and over a quarter reported that siblings were rarely or never helpful. While in some cases brothers and sisters rallied support around the time of husbands' deaths, this support tended to dwindle as the years went by. Siblings returned to their own homes and their own lives once the crisis had passed. By the time of the interviews, brothers and sisters played a relatively minor role as sources of economic aid, services, companionship, or emotional support, especially when compared to the help given by adult children.

In contrast to Lopata, Shanas (1979, 1980) highlights the extent to which many siblings remain in contact with one another and serve as sources of support in times of need. She reports that about one-third of the elderly respondents surveyed had seen a sibling during the past week, and three-quarters of those who had never married had visited with a brother or sister in the last seven days. Moreover, Shanas contends that "widowed persons and older persons who have never married are especially dependent on their brothers and sisters. For many widowed persons, siblings assume some of the responsibilities of a now deceased husband or wife. Many persons who have never married live in the same household with a sibling" (p. 7). While adult children may provide more support, the sibling bond should not be discounted, especially for those elderly without children or spouses.

Whereas Lopata stresses the relative absence of siblings in the support systems of older women, Shanas emphasizes the extent to which they are present. Neither analysis, however, pays much attention to the ways in which sibling relations are socially patterned. Research by Cantor (1979) suggests that both the proximity of siblings and the frequency of interaction are shaped by older people's social class backgrounds, ethnicity, and gender. Within her sample of generally low-income elderly living in New York's inner city, women, Hispanics, and more affluent respondents were more likely to have a brother or sister living nearby and to interact with that sibling on a regular basis. Aside from this work, however, there is little recent information on how social characteristics and life histories of the elderly affect how much help is given to or received from siblings in old age. Nor is much known about what older people expect in the way of service exchanges with siblings or how satisfied they are with the support they do give and receive. This is one sphere of family relations that clearly warrants further research.

Ties to Younger Generations

Although relationships between parents and adult children generally extend over several decades, much of the research on this intergenerational tie has focused on events and circumstances occurring at the beginning or end of the adult life cycle—family formation on the part of the young adult children and illness and infirmity on the part of the parents (e.g., Adams, 1968; Cicirelli, 1981; Hill et al., 1970; Robinson and Thurnher, 1979; Sussman and Burchinal, 1962). In doing so, such studies yield an image of intergenerational help patterns that is basically asymmetric over the adult life course. Parents give more to adult children than they receive when offspring are young and receive more than they give when they themselves are old. While not an inaccurate portrayal of the overall flow of assistance, this characterization understates the extent to which elderly parents continue to provide support to their mid-life children. Based on results from a 1975 national survey, Shanas (1980) notes that although seven out of ten elderly respondents reported receiving aid from their children, a similar proportion reported giving assistance as well. Similarly, while 87% of the low-income elderly interviewed by Cantor (1979) reported getting assistance from offspring, three-quarters had rendered some form of help.

The types of assistance typically provided by elderly parents include gifts, help during illness and other emergencies, babysitting and the like. In Cantor's (1979) survey about two-thirds of the elderly respondents reported giving monetary gifts or presents to their children and about half reported stepping in during times of illness. Estimates of babysitting and child care vary widely from study to study and probably reflect differences in question wording (e.g., occasional babysitting versus regular child care) as well as differences in the ages and proximity of children and the ages and health of grandparents. For example, Lopata (1979) reports that about one-fifth of the widows interviewed ''help(ed) take care of children''; Guttmann (1979) states that about one-third of his white ethnic sample of elderly reported babysitting for their families, while 92% of the grandmothers interviewed by Robertson (1977) reported some babysitting and over half (55%) babysat at least once a month. Family businesses remain common in some ethnic groups (e.g., Jewish, Italian, and Japanese-American), with occupational skills and ownership often passing from fathers to sons (Woehrer, 1978).

In addition to these very tangible forms of aid are the less tangible ways that elderly parents contribute to the well-being of their children. In some families, elderly mothers remain the focal point of extended kinship activities, convening family rituals, orchestrating holidays, and making sure that family members keep in touch. Martin and Martin (1978), for example, highlight the role of elderly widows in many black extended families. Summarizing the results of Martin and Martin's study, Streib and Beck (1980) write,

> these important persons (elderly black widows) act as communication centers for the family: They direct family celebrations, help socialize the children, define what constitutes deviant behavior, and help arbitrate family conflicts. This role of elderly women in strengthening families' capabilities to meet crises and difficulties is striking, for their efforts are directed to enhancing the welfare of others, not primarily to insuring their own welfare. (p. 948)

While most elderly parents report helping their children in some capacity, this does not necessarily mean that their support is forthcoming regularly and frequently. Research on family help patterns, in fact, suggests that there are wide variations in the amounts and types of aid extended and in the degree to which elderly parents remain a part of their children's daily lives. Help patterns are not only influenced by such obvious factors as proximity and parental health but also by the needs of children, the resources of parents, and family norms about generational autonomy and closeness. Based on her study of New York's inner-city elderly, Cantor (1979), for example, reports that black and Hispanic elderly provided more assistance and were generally more involved with their children than elderly white respondents. She speculates that this greater involvement and aid reflect "both the greater presence of the extended family in the Hispanic community and the greater need among low-income minority groups for intergenerational assistance as a means of offsetting the effects of poverty and discrimination" (p. 169). In addition to income, Stueve and Lein (1979) suggest that the life stage of children affects the flow of assistance from parents to offspring. As children grow older, become more financially secure, and move beyond the early child-rearing years, many no longer seem to need the tangible aid that parents once provided.

The value families place on generational independence also shapes patterns of help. In her review of the literature on ethnicity and aging, Woehrer (1978) notes that ethnic groups differ in how strictly they perceive boundaries between nuclear family units. She suggests that "whereas a German or Scandinavian American may perceive carefully defined boundaries around the nuclear families of her children, those boundaries may be much more vague for a black grandmother. Thus, while the German grandmother may not view it as in her place to give advice or rear her grandchildren, the black grandmother may very well perceive it as her responsibility to rear a grandchild, or a niece or nephew, or to give advice and assistance in rearing the children of her kin" (p. 333; see also Guttmann, 1979). Differences have also been noted between working- and middle-class families, with greater physical and emotional separation characterizing more affluent generations (Cantor, 1979; Troll et al., 1979).

The research discussed above is based primarily on self-reports by the older generation; much less is known about how mid-life children view their parents' efforts to provide help. While much aid is undoubtedly appreciated, research by Wilcox (1981) suggests that help and assistance can be a two-edged sword. In his study of individuals' adjustment to divorce, he found that whereas family members were the most supportive people following a divorce, they were also the most judgmental. Efforts to aid can also be experienced as attempts at intrusion. There has also been little research on the extent to which elderly parents enhance the psychological well-being and morale of children, although there have been many studies of children's effects on parents (e.g., Arling, 1976; Duff and Hong, 1980; Larson, 1978; Liang et al., 1980; Seelbach and Sauer, 1977). One exception is research by Baruch and Barnett (1981) on the concerns and gratifications experienced by approximately 300 mid-life women (ages 35 to 55). Although the ages of mothers and class backgrounds of daughters are not specified, they report that most mid-life women interviewed found their relationships with mothers rewarding and that many looked to their mothers as "reassuring role model(s) of the aging process." Moreover, having a rewarding mother-daughter relationship seemed to heighten a sense of mastery and life satisfaction on the part of women who were not mothers themselves. The authors suggest that perhaps relationships with mothers take on greater significance for women who maintain few social roles and intimate associations. To date, much of the literature on children's perceptions of elderly parents has focused on the problems and difficulties children encounter when parents become needy or dependent. While dependency can certainly place constraints on children's lives, research such as that by Baruch and Barnett indicates that greater attention should be paid to the positive ways elderly parents affect offspring as well.

In concluding this section, it should be noted that providing support to offspring is not without costs. Anecdotal and ethnographic accounts which focus on the process of intergenerational exchange (e.g., Matthews, 1979; Sherudi, 1979) indicate that in extending offers of help, parents can become enmeshed in difficult interpersonal encounters with their adult children. For example, one issue that has surfaced in both academic and popular writing is the resentment many older people express when children's expectations for support exceed the level that parents want to provide (e.g., Colher and Grunebaum, 1981; Sherudi, 1979). If parents refuse their offspring, children may feel rebuffed and deprived of legitimate help; if they acquiesce, parents may come to resent what are seen as repeated and inconvenient intrusions on their time. Other difficulties stem from differing notions of what parents can rightfully expect from children when they offer support. Matthews (1979), for example, provides some evidence that older mothers feel angry and slighted when offspring willingly accept their material help but reject their efforts to offer advice. Even more problematic may be those situations in which older mothers want to participate in children's lives but are limited by offspring to sporadic contact or ritualized roles (ibid.). Aside from such anecdotal accounts, however, little is known about the extent to which older parents experience such difficulties in their role as support providers or the ways in which interpersonal tensions are handled and resolved.

Grandchildren and great-grandchildren. Perhaps it is in their role as grandparents that older people are most often portrayed as positive contributors to family life, especially to the well-being of children. Many children's books (e.g., Brandenberg, 1979; Greenfield, 1980) as well as several popular discussions of grandparenting (e.g., Shedd, 1976) depict the grandparent-grandchild tie as a special bond, a private, intimate, one-to-one relationship that is cherished by both old and young. Some of the clinical literature on intergenerational relations echoes a similar theme. Kornhaber and Woodward (1981), for example, argue that:

> emotional attachments between grandparents and grandchildren are unique. The normal conflicts that occur between children and parents simply do not exist between grandchildren and grandparents. This is because grandparents, no mat-

ter what they were like as parents, are exempt from the emotional intensity that characterizes parent-child relationships.
. . . In short, grandparents and grandchildren do not have to do
anything to make each other happy. Their happiness comes
from being together. (p. xiii)

While there has been an upsurge of popular and clinical writing
on grandparenting in recent years, researchers have been slow to
investigate this tie. As a result, research findings on grandparents
and grandchildren are limited and scattered. In general, interviews
with grandparents and young adult grandchildren tend to support
the view that older people play a largely emotional or expressive
role in grandchildren's lives (e.g., McDonald and Hagestad, 1979;
Neugarten and Weinstein, 1964; Robertson, 1976, 1977); they are
more likely to be sources of emotional gratification and companionship than instrumental support and advice. There is also some
indirect evidence that contact with grandparents has a positive influence on young children. Kornhaber and Woodward (1981) interviewed approximately 300 children between the ages of five and
eighteen and asked them to draw pictures of their grandparents.
Based on a thematic analysis of the children's drawings and com-
ments, they maintain that frequent contact with grandparents not
only enriches the emotional lives of youngsters but also provides
them with connections to the past and role models for the future.
In a different vein, Troll et al. (1979) review research suggesting
that children with grandparents and great-grandparents tend to be
more accepting of old people and show fewer signs of age-pre-
judice. Aside from these studies, however, there has been little research on the evolution of the grandparent-grandchild tie or on the
effects of grandparents on children's development.

While the grandparent-grandchild tie is often described as a special bond, little is also known about the extent to which older people form such ties. The few available estimates vary widely and
are based on different samples and measures. Kornhaber and
Woodward (1981) report that the vast majority (95%) of the 300 or
so grandparents they interviewed maintained at best sporadic contact with grandchildren. However, since their sample was not
drawn in a random or systematic manner, it is unknown how accurately it reflects the population at large; moreover, what is meant
by sporadic contact is unclear. Two other studies, one based on a
largely working-class sample of 125 grandmothers (Robertson,
1977) and the other based on a middle-class sample of 70 couples

(Neugarten and Weinstein, 1964) found that about one-fourth of the respondents remained distant figures in grandchildren's lives. What is significant about the latter two studies, however, is that older grandparents were less likely to maintain distant relationships and more likely to get involved with grandchildren than middle-aged grandparents, perhaps because this older generation has stronger extended family orientations, perhaps because they have fewer midlife commitments, such as employment and community activities.

Developing a close relation with grandchildren and seeing them often is not simply a matter of geographic proximity; all of the distant grandparents interviewed by Neugarten and Weinstein (1964) lived in the same metropolitan area as at least one grandchild. Other factors such as the life-styles and preferences of grandparents also affect older people's interactions with the young. Not all elderly, for example, enjoy spending time with children, and many have other employment, family, and community involvements that occupy their time (Robertson, 1977). In addition, both research and anecdotal accounts suggest that the middle generation of parents sometimes acts as gatekeepers to children. Where ties between older people and their adult children are tenuous, contact with younger generations may be limited (e.g., Sherudi, 1979; Troll et al., 1979). Divorce on the part of the middle generation can also sever bonds, especially between paternal grandparents and grandchildren. Unlike fathers, grandparents have no legal rights to visit with grandchildren.

The discussion above has focused on the ways older people are involved with grandchildren during the first half of the grandparenting career. With greater longevity, however, growing numbers of elderly not only have middle-aged grandchildren but great-grandchildren and great-great-grandchildren as well. To date, virtually nothing is known about these relationships. While we might suspect that older people who have maintained minimal contact with young grandchildren will invest little emotional energy in these ties, it is unclear how older people who take an active stance towards grandparenting will respond to these new roles. Such analysis awaits the future.

THE ELDERLY AS PARTICIPANTS IN EXTRA-FAMILIAL NETWORKS AND THE WIDER COMMUNITY

While the family constitutes an important locus of interaction for many elderly, especially for those from working-class and certain ethnic backgrounds, it is by no means the only arena in which older people play an active role. Friendships, neighborly relations, volunteer work, and voluntary associations act as other outlets for the time, energy, and contributions of older men and women. This section examines such extra-familial involvements, beginning with those informal ties in which older people may give as much as they receive and then turning to ways older people become involved in their communities.

Informal Ties to Neighbors and Friends

Friendships and neighboring ties among the old are usually conceptualized as voluntary relationships based on balanced reciprocity (e.g., Arling, 1976; Hochschild, 1973; Wentowski, 1979). Unlike the more obligatory and sometimes unequal exchanges that characterize kinship ties, these relationships are built on the premise that both parties will contribute about as much as they receive. In engaging in such relationships, elderly people tacitly agree to become sources of companionship and support as well as recipients.

While these informal ties tend to be reciprocal in nature, ethnographic accounts indicate that older people vary considerably in what they consider to be appropriate exchanges with neighbors and friends and in the extent to which they become enmeshed in extra-familial ties. At one extreme are the multi-dimensional relationships and personal communities that sometimes develop in age-segregated settings, where elderly neighbors become friends and where elderly friends not only engage in frequent socializing but also share sentiments, provide intimacy, and cooperate in systems of mutual help (e.g., Hochschild, 1973). At the other extreme are the marginal ties that characterize many elderly residents of inner-city hotels and single-room lodgings (e.g., Eckert, 1977; Stephens, 1976). Among this population, entangling exchanges are avoided and self-reliance is stressed, and yet, even here, elderly residents are likely to look out for one another and come to each others' aid in the case of emergencies. As Hess (1976) points out, most elderly fall somewhere in-between these two extremes in the extent to which they participate with neighbors and friends in the give and take of mutual support.

Anthropological research by Wentowski (1979) points to the importance of personal styles in shaping how older persons define their neighboring and friendship relations. Although the older people she interviewed expressed a desire to live on their own and maintain their independence, they differed in the strategies adopted to achieve this end. While some preferred to gamble on their ability to remain self-reliant, others preferred to invest time and energy into constructing neighboring and friendship relationships based on mutual help. In addition to variations in personal styles, expectations about friendships and neighboring relations are grounded in cultural beliefs which are passed from one generation to the next. Hess (1979) argues that persistent gender differences in friendship patterns (in particular, the greater propensity of females of all ages to engage in intimate friendships and self-disclosure) are closely linked to sex-role learning and expectations. Characteristics of residential communities also affect extra-familial ties, especially the extent to which older residents come to think of neighbors as more than the people who, by chance, live next door. Since friendships and neighborly relations tend to be based on reciprocity, they are more likely to develop in settings where people share similar interests and concerns. Several studies indicate that age-segregated housing tends to promote friendship formation and interaction between older people and their neighbors (e.g., Hochschild, 1973; Rosow, 1967), although research by Sherman (1975a, b) and Jacobs (1975) shows that age-similarity alone is not sufficient to insure close ties. Finally, as might be expected, both the desire and opportunity to interact with neighbors and friends are shaped by the elderly's access to such resources as good health, transportation, income, and the like (see reviews by Chown, 1981; Hess, 1976, Lowenthal and Robinson, 1976). More affluent and healthy elderly, for example, are less likely to form close associates in the neighborhood, in part because they have the wherewithal to look elsewhere for friends (Rosow, 1967; Sherman, 1975).

While most older people engage in some form of neighboring or friendship activity, research on the content of these relations— what is actually exchanged between neighbors and friends—is relatively scarce. Although most older people, like younger adults, live in age-integrated communities, much of the ethnographic work on informal exchanges focuses on age-segregated settings (e.g., Hochschild, 1973; Jacobs, 1975; Johnson, 1971) or "problem" populations. Surveys focus on more representative samples, but they often overlook the content of neighboring and friendship relations and are limited to an examination of such structural features as the number of ties, frequency of contact, age and sex similarity, and the like (e.g., Booth and Hess, 1974; Petrowsky, 1976; Powers and Bultena, 1976). Surveys tend to look at how often people see their friends but not how they define or value the friendship relation. These research limitations are both surprising and unfortunate given the important role that friendship and neighboring ties play in enhancing the life satisfaction and well-being of the old (e.g., Arling, 1976; Blau, 1973). In particular, further research is needed which examines how the content and meaning of friendship change over the life course, how definitions of friendship and neighboring relations vary within the elderly population, and how extra-familial relations with age-peers differ from those between young and old.

The Elderly as Members of their Communities

Along with their involvements in the give and take of personal relations, a sizeable minority of elderly are engaged in more direct forms of community service through their efforts as volunteers. Results from two national surveys estimate that between 14% and 22% of the elderly participate in some form of volunteer activity, while an additional 10% express interest in doing so (Action, 1974; Harris and Associates, 1975). In addition to activities generally thought of as "volunteer work," the majority of elderly (between 70% and 80%) also participate in some form of voluntary association, such as churches, fraternal and ethnic organizations, and veterans groups (Babchuk and Booth, 1969; Babchuk et al., 1979; Cutler, 1976a). Finally, in some cases elderly come to be known as "natural helpers" by people in their communities or participate in a variety of self-help groups.

Although the elderly are not often though of as volunteers, their visibility has been heightened in recent years both by the Reagan administration's promotion of Foster Grandparents as a model program of volunteer service and by the emergence over the last two decades of volunteer programs designed specifically to tap the time and skills of this older age group. Programs such as SERVE and RSVP act as umbrella organizations which recruit, train, and place elderly volunteers in a variety of community institutions ranging from schools and libraries to nursing homes and hospitals (Sainer, 1976). Created by federal legislation in 1969, RSVP had established programs in nearly 700 communities using over 165,000 elderly participants by the mid-1970s (ibid.). Although often set up as social and recreational programs, many senior centers have also become focal points for volunteer work entailing service delivery to the old (e.g., Payne, 1977).

Despite their growing visibility, much remains to be learned about the characteristics of older volunteers. For example, although it is often assumed that volunteers tend to be drawn from young, healthier, and more affluent segments of the elderly population, project descriptions indicate that at least some organizations are effective in utilizing the skills of less advantaged groups. Sainer (1976), for example, reports that in the case of SERVE, it was the oldest volunteers "who undertook the largest number of assignments and contributed the greatest number of hours of service" (p. 73). Moreover, she notes that SERVE has also been successful in recruiting elderly with limited incomes and educations as well as in developing projects which draw upon the services of such groups as the blind and nursing home residents. Similarly, although volunteer work has been promoted as a new role for late life, there is little information on the prior involvements of elderly volunteers. For example, it is not known whether most elderly participants are first-time volunteers or life-long contributors. Since much of the information on older volunteers is based on case studies of particular programs, it is not surprising that participant profiles vary from study to study. Comparative analyses are needed in order to identify both what types of people are most likely to volunteer their time and what it is about different programs (e.g., their recruiting procedures, the nature of volunteer activities, the characteristics of the community served) that affects their ability to recruit and keep older participants.

There is also much to be learned regarding the benefits of volunteer work, for example, the extent to which it constitutes meaningful work for the old. Payne (1977), among others, has described the volunteer role as a potential "intervention strategy which may provide role continuity, satisfaction, enhancement of the self-concept, and social support systems" (p. 355), yet there have been few efforts to document this claim. Although it is not surprising that older volunteers tend to report satisfaction with the role (otherwise they would presumably terminate their involvement), there is little information on what types of activities are regarded as most rewarding or on the extent to which older volunteers would prefer to be involved in paid, rather than unpaid, work. Similarly, research on the performance of older volunteers is limited. One exception is an early evaluation of the Foster Grandparent program, which documented the positive effects of older volunteers on the social and cognitive development of children (Saltz, 1970). Other volunteer programs warrant similar attention.

On a more practical note, several case studies provide useful information on circumstances that can hinder the participation of older volunteers. Sainer (1976) highlights the importance of incorporating transportation arrangements into volunteer programs since many elderly do not drive, making travel to agencies expensive, tiring, or simply inconvenient. Faulkner (1975) emphasizes the importance of considering the physical safety of participants, especially when programs are located in inner-city areas; she describes how one agency was forced to rethink its proposal to use elderly blacks as informal outreach workers when it became clear that their safety could not be assured.

The above discussion focuses on the more structured forms of volunteer work. In addition to this type of work, some elderly also participate in more indigenous forms of help-giving. Research by Patterson (1977) points out that some elderly act as "natural helpers," that is, people to whom others "turn naturally in time of trouble or difficulty" (p. 161). Unaffiliated with any organizations, they become known in their immediate communities as people who are able and willing to help with a variety of problems, from listening to the marital difficulties of a neighbor to providing transportation and companionship to an elderly widow from their church. In her study of indigenous help-giving in several rural communities, Patterson found that the elderly comprised about one-third of all the natural helpers identified by local residents. These older natural helpers varied considerably in terms of their educational and occupational backgrounds, but were similar in two respects. First, they expressed a similar openness to helping others and an ease with offering non-professional advice. Second, they saw helping as part of their lives—they did not see themselves as "natural helpers" even though others in the community did so (Patterson, 1977; Patterson and Twente, 1971).

While the emphasis is on helping others in the case of natural helpers and formal volunteers, the elderly also join together to provide mutual help and support. With the increasing recognition of the effectiveness of peer-support groups in easing life transitions and dealing with many of the problems of both young and old, a number of programs serving the elderly have emerged. Perhaps the most widespread and publicized program is Widows-to-Widows, a community-based system of peer counseling which has two purposes. It both provides the recently widowed with the help and support needed throughout the early stages of grief and sets in motion the development of new relationships which may persist beyond the lifetime of any particular group.

Not all self-help groups are focused on the life crises of individuals. A number of groups have emerged whose purpose is to better the welfare of the elderly at large. The National Council of Senior Citizens, for example, was originally formed to lobby for Medicare and now campaigns for a whole array of elderly concerns (Pratt, 1976). Other such groups include the National Retired Teachers Association—American Association of Retired Persons (NRTA-AARP), the National Association of Federal Employees (NARFE), and the Gray Panthers. The NRTA-AARP alone reports over nine million members, making it one of the largest voluntary organizations in the nation (Pratt, 1977).

While a substantial number of the elderly are involved in such age-based organizations, they are by no means the most common form of membership. Like people of all ages, the old are most likely to belong to church-affiliated groups (Cutler, 1976b); fraternal and veterans organizations also draw large numbers of the old (ibid.). Those who belong to such voluntary associations have typically been joiners throughout their lives (Lowenthal and Robinson, 1976). There is little evidence that participation declines dramatically in old age (Babchuk and Booth, 1969; Babchuk et al., 1979; Cutler, 1977) and little evidence that older people join groups as a way of compensating for other age-related losses.

As this section has indicated, there is a diversity of ways the elderly can be involved in their communities, as neighbors, natural helpers, peer-counselors, volunteer workers, church-goers, senior-center members, Gray Panthers, and the like. The evidence accummulated to date on these forms of participation combats the image of older people as withdrawing from social relations and becoming passive members of their communities. For the overwhelming proportion of their lives, the elderly clearly remain active in the give and take of community life, just as they remain active in the more intimate world of family and friends.

CONCLUSION

Researchers have looked at the social relations of the old through many lenses, but most have come away with an image of the elderly's social worlds as contracting and of the elderly as withdrawing from many forms of community life. Disengagement theorists Cumming and Henry (1961), for example, noted a tendency on the part of Kansas City adults to withdraw from social involvements as they grew older and interpreted this behavior as a normal life-course occurrence, a developmental phenomenon that is beneficial to both individuals and society. Activity theorists also acknowledge a general decline in social participation but view this decline as neither natural nor beneficial. More often than not, "modern society" is blamed for excluding the elderly and for underutilizing the talents of the old. More recently, social scientists have drawn upon exchange and power theories to account for the elderly's waning involvements (e.g., Dowd, 1975). The elderly are portrayed as a disadvantaged age group which lacks the power and resources to engage in favorable social exchanges. Having little of value to offer other generations, the elderly are either cast into dependent relations or pressed to withdraw from social ties.

While acknowledging that constraints on social participation increase in old age, especially with the onset of illness, disabilities, death of friends, and the like, this paper has examined the networks of the elderly from a different standpoint and emphasized the many ways that older adults remain active in their families, neighborhoods, and wider communities. Although it is not surprising to learn that most older people continue to participate in the give and take of social relations, examining the ways they contribute to their social worlds is important for several reasons. First, it makes clear that images of dependency, passivity, and declining participation at best characterize only a portion of the later years. Throughout much of old age, most people are healthy and socially involved. Focusing on older people as active network members also reminds us that the elderly are a diverse population. While there may be some common decline in social participation in advanced old age, the elderly clearly differ in how they construct their social worlds and how they define and value personal relations. These differences reflect not only variations among the old in their current situations but also lifelong differences in personal backgrounds and styles. Finally, the evidence accumulated here clearly indicates that although power and resources may decrease in old age, many elderly still have much to offer age peers and other generations in their roles as family members, friends, neighbors, natural helpers, and volunteers.

Although there are sizeable literatures on the kinship, friendship, and community involvements of the elderly, much remains to be learned about older people's participation in social worlds. Many specific examples of needed research have been indicated throughout this review, but one issue warrants special mention. To date, much of the research has focused on one or two types of personal relations but has paid little attention to how social ties fit together to form social worlds, for example, how involvement in family activities affects investment in friendships or how public and private spheres intersect. People's social networks are a composite of many different kinds of relationships. Understanding how these different commitments are packaged and managed remains an important task for future research.

REFERENCES

Action. *Americans volunteer*. Washington, 1974.

Adams, B. N. *Kinship in an urban setting*. Chicago: Markham, 1968.

Archbold, P. G. Impact of caring for an ill elderly parent on the middle-aged or elderly offspring caregiver. Paper presented at the 31st Annual Scientific Meeting of the Gerontological Society of America, Dallas, November 1978.

Arling, G. The elderly widow and her family, neighbors and friends. *Journal of Marriage and the Family*, 1976, *38*, 757–768.

Atchley, R. C., and Miller, S. J. Older people and their families. In C. Eisdorfer et al. (Eds.), *Annual review of gerontology and geriatrics*, Vol. 1. New York: Springer, 1980.

Babchuk, N., and Booth, A. Voluntary association memberships: A longitudinal analysis. *American Sociological Review*, 1969, *34*, 31–45.

Babchuk, N., Peters, G. R., Hoyt, D. R., and Kaiser, M. A. The voluntary associations of the aged. *Journal of Gerontology*, 1979, *34*, 579–587.

Baruch, G., and Barnett, R. C. Adult daughters' relationships with their mothers: The era of good feelings. Working Paper No. 74, Wellesley College Center for Research on Women, 1981.

Blau, Z. S. *Old age in a changing society*. New York: Franklin Watts, 1973.

Booth, A., and Hess, E. Cross-sex friendships. *Journal of Marriage and the Family*, 1974, *36*, 38–47.

Branch, L. G. *Understanding the health and social service needs of people over age 65*. Center for Survey Research, University of Massachusetts and the Joint Center for Urban Studies of MIT and Harvard University, 1977.

Brandenberg, A. *The two of them*. New York: Greenwillow Books, 1979.

Brody, E. M. Aged parents and aging children. In P. K. Ragan (Ed.), *Aging parents*. Los Angeles: The Ethel Percy Andrus Gerontology Center, 1979.

Brody, S., Poulschock, W., and Masciocchi, C. The family caring unit: A major consideration in the long-term support system. *The Gerontologist,* 1978, *18,* 556–561.

Brown, B. B. The impact of confidants on adjustment to stressful events in adulthood. Paper presented at the 33rd Annual Scientific Meeting of the Gerontological Society of America, San Diego, November 1980.

Bultena, G. L., and Powers, E. A. Denial of aging: Age identification and reference group orientations. *Journal of Gerontology,* 1978, *33,* 748–754.

Cantor, M. H. Neighbors and friends: An overlooked resource in the informal support system. Paper presented at the 30th Annual Scientific Meeting of the Gerontological Society of America, San Francisco, November 1977.

Cantor, M. H. The informal support system of New York's inner city elderly: Is ethnicity a factor? In D. E. Gelfand and A. J. Kutzik (Eds.), *Ethnicity and aging.* New York: Springer, 1979.

Cantor, M. H. Caring for the frail elderly: Impact on family, friends, and neighbors. Paper presented at the 33rd Annual Scientific Meeting of the Gerontological Society of America, San Diego, November 1980.

Chown, S. M. Friendship in old age. In S. Duck and R. Gilmour (Eds.), *Personal relationships 2: Developing personal relationships.* New York: Academic Press, 1981.

Cicirelli, V. G. *Helping elderly parents.* Boston: Auburn House, 1981.

Coehn, S. Z., and Gans, B. M. *The other generation gap.* Chicago: Follett, 1978.

Cohler, B. J., and Grunebaum, H. U. *Mothers, grandmothers, and daughters.* New York: John Wiley & Sons, 1981.

Cohler, B. J., and Lieberman, M. A. Personality change across the second half of life: Findings from a study of Irish, Italian, and Polish-American men and women. In D. E. Gelfand and A. J. Kutzik (Eds.), *Ethnicity and aging.* New York: Springer, 1979.

Crossman, L., London, D., and Barry, C. Older women caring for disabled spouses: A model for supportive services. *The Gerontologist,* 1981, *21,* 464–470.

Cumming, E., and Henry W. *Growing old.* New York: Basic Books, 1961.

Cutler, S. J. Membership in different types of voluntary associations and psychological well-being. *The Gerontologist,* 1976, *16,* 335–339.

Cutler, S. J. Age profiles of membership in sixteen types of voluntary associations. *Journal of Gerontology,* 1976, *31,* 462–470.

Cutler, S. J. Aging and voluntary association participation. *Journal of Gerontology,* 1977, *32,* 470–479.

Dowd, J. J. Aging as an exchange: A preface to theory. *Journal of Gerontology,* 1975, *30,* 584–594.

Duff, R. W., and Hong, L. K. Quality and quantity of social interactions in the life satisfaction of older Americans. Unpublished manuscript, 1980.

Eckert, J. K. Health status, adjustments, and social supports of older people living in center city hotels. Paper presented at the 30th Annual Scientific Meeting of the Gerontological Society of America, San Francisco, November 1977.

Faulkner, A. O. The black aged as good neighbors: An experiment in volunteer service. *The Gerontologist,* 1975, *15,* 554–559.

Feldman, H. Development of the husband-wife relationship. Preliminary report, Cornell Studies of Marital Development: Study in the Transition to Parenthood. Department of Child Development and Family Relationships. New York State College of Home Economics, Cornell University, 1964.

Fengler, A., and Goodrich, N. Wives of elderly disabled men: The hidden victims. *The Gerontologist,* 1979, *19,* 175–183.

Fischer, C. S., and Phillips, S. L. "Who is alone?" Social characteristics of people with small networks. Working paper No. 310, University of California (Berkeley) Institute of Urban and Regional Development, 1979.

Greenfield, E. *Grandmama's joy.* New York and Cleveland: Collins, 1980.

Guttmann, D. Use of informal and formal supports by white ethnic aged. In D. E. Gelfand and A. J. Kutzik (Eds.), *Ethnicity and aging.* New York: Springer, 1979.

Harris, L. and Associates. *The myth and reality of aging in America.* Washington, DC: National Council on Aging, Inc, 1975.

Hess, B. B. Sex roles, friendship, and the life course. *Research on Aging,* 1979, *1,* 494–515.

Hess, B. H. Self-help among the aged. *Social Policy,* 1976, *7,* 55–62.

Hill, R., Foote, N., Aldous, J. Carlson, R., and MacDonald, R. *Family development in three generations.* Cambridge, MA: Schenkman, 1970.

Hochschild, A. R. *The unexpected community.* Englewood Cliffs, NJ: Prentice-Hall, 1973.

Hutchison, I. W., III. The significance of marital status for morale and life satisfaction among lower-income elderly. *Journal of Marriage and the Family,* 1975, *37,* 287–293.

Isaacs, B., Livingstone, M., and Neville, Y. *Survival of the unfittest.* London: Routledge and Kegan Paul, 1972.

Jacobs, J. *Older persons and retirement communities.* Springfield, IL: Charles C. Thomas, 1975.

Johnson, C. L. Obligation and reciprocity in caregiving during illness: A comparison of spouses and offspring as family supports. Paper presented at the 33rd Annual Scientific Meeting of the Gerontological Society of America, San Diego, November 1980.

Johnson, S. K. *Idle haven: Community building among the working-class retired.* Berkeley, CA: University of California Press, 1971.

Kerckhoff, A. C. Family patterns and morale in retirement. In I. H. Simpson and J. C. McKinney (Eds.), *Social aspects of aging.* Durham, NC: Duke University Press, 1966.

Kornhaber, A., and Woodward, K. *Grandparents/Grandchildren: The vital connection.* Garden City, NY: Anchor Press/Doubleday, 1981.

Kovar, M. G. Elderly people: The population 65 years and over. In *Health, United States: 1976–1977,* National Center for Health Statistics, Washington, DC: U.S. Government Printing Office, 1977.

Larson, R. Thirty years of research on the subjective well-being of older Americans. *Journal of Gerontology,* 1978, *33,* 109–125.

Lewis, M. A., Bienenstock, R., Cantor, M., and Schneewind, E. The extent to which informal and formal supports interact to maintain the older people in the community. Paper presented at the 33rd Annual Scientific Meeting of the Gerontological Society of America, San Diego, November 1980.

Liang, J., Dvorkin, L., Kahana, E., and Mazian, F. Social integration and morale: A re-examination. *Journal of Gerontology,* 1980, *35,* 746–757.

Lopata, H. Z. *Widowhood in an American city.* Cambridge, MA: Schenkman, 1973.

Lopata, H. Z. *Women as widows: Support systems.* New York: Elsevier-North Holland, 1979.

Lowenthal, M. F., and Haven, C. Interaction and adaptation: Intimacy as a critical variable. *American Sociological Review,* 1968, *33,* 20–30.

Lowenthal, M. F., and Robinson, B. Social networks and isolation. In R. H. Binstock and E. Shanas (Eds.), *Handbook of aging and the social sciences.* New York: Van Nostrand Reinhold Company, 1976.

Lutsky, N. S. Attitudes toward old age and elderly persons. In C. Eisdorfer et al. (Eds.), *Annual review of gerontology and geriatrics,* Vol. I. New York: Springer, 1980.

Martin, E. P., and Martin, J. *The Black extended family.* Chicago: University of Chicago Press, 1978.

Matthews, S. H. *The social world of old women.* Beverly Hills, CA: Sage Publications, 1979.

McDonald, M. V., and Hagestad, G. O. Perceptions of grandparents by their adult grandchildren. Paper presented at the 30th Annual Scientific Meeting of the Gerontological Society of America, San Francisco, November 1977.

Miller, S. J. Widowhood and the older woman. Paper presented at the 30th Annual Scientific Meeting of the Gerontological Society of America, San Francisco, November 1977.

Morgan, L. A. Problems of widowhood. In P. K. Ragan (Ed.), *Aging parents.* Los Angeles: The Ethel Percy Andrus Gerontology Center, 1979.

Neugarten, B. and Associates. *Personality in middle and late life.* New York: Atherton, 1964.

Neugarten, B. Personality change in late life: A developmental perspective. In C. Eisdorfer and M. P. Lawton (Eds.), *The psychology of adult development and aging.* Washington, DC: American Psychological Association, 1973.

Neugarten, B. The middle generations. In P. K. Ragan (Ed.), *Aging parents.* Los Angeles: The Ethel Percy Andrus Gerontology Center, 1979.

Neugarten, B., and Weinstein, K. The changing American grandparent. *Journal of Marriage and the Family,* 1964, *26,* 199–204.

Orthner, D. K. Leisure activity patterns and marital satisfaction over the marital career. *Journal of Marriage and the Famly,* 1975, *37,* 91–102.

Patterson, S. L. Toward a conceptualization of natural helping. *Arete,* 1977, *4,* 161–173.

Patterson, S. L., and Twente, E. E. Older natural helpers: Their characteristics and patterns of helping. *Public Welfare,* 1971, *29,* 400–403.

Payne, B. P. The older volunteers: Social role continuity and development. *The Gerontologist,* 1977, *17,* 355–361.

Petrowsky, M. Marital status, sex, and the social networks of the elderly. *Journal of Marriage and the Family,* 1976, *38,* 747–756.

Pilisuk, M., and Minkler, M. Supportive networks: Life ties for the elderly. *The Journal of Social Issues,* 1980, *36,* 95–116.

Powers, E. A., and Bultena, G. L. Sex differences in intimate friendships of old age. *Journal of Marriage and the Family,* 1976, *38,* 739–747.

Pratt, H. J. *The gray lobby.* Chicago: University of Chicago Press, 1976.

Raskind, M. A., and Storric, M. G. The organic mental disorders. In E. W. Busse and D. G. Blazer (Eds.), *Handbook of geriatric psychiatry.* New York: Van Nostrand Reinhold, 1980.

Robertson, J. F. Significance of grandparents: Perceptions of young adult grandchildren. *The Gerontologist,* 1976, *16,* 137–140.

Robertson, J. F. Grandmotherhood: A study of role conceptions. *Journal of Marriage and the Family,* 1977, *39,* 165–174.

Robinson, B., and Thurnher, M. Taking care of aged parents: A family cycle transition. *The Gerontologist,* 1979, *19,* 586–593.

Rollins, B. C., and Cannon, K. L. Marital satisfaction over the family life cycle: A reevaluation. *Journal of Marriage and the Family,* 1974, *35,* 271–282.

Rosow, I. *Social integration of the aged.* New York: Free Press, 1967.

Sainer, J. S. The community cares: Older volunteers. *Social Policy,* 1976, *7,* 73–75.

Saltz, R. Evaluation of a foster-grandparent program. In A. Kadushin (Ed.), *Child welfare services: A sourcebook.* New York: Macmillan, 1970.

Schwartz, A. N. *Survival handbook for children of aging parents.* Chicago: Follett, 1977.

Seelbach, W. C., and Sauer, W. J. Filial responsibility expectations and morale among aged parents. *The Gerontologist,* 1977, *17,* 492-499.

Shanas, E. The family as social support system in old age. Paper presented at the 30th Annual Scientific Meeting of the Gerontological Society of America, San Francisco, November 1977.

Shanas, E. Social myth as hypothesis: The case of the family relations of old people. *The Gerontologist,* 1979, *19,* 3–9.

Shanas, E. The family as social support system in old age. *The Gerontologist,* 1979, *19,* 169–174.

Shanas, E. Older people and their families: The new pioneers. *Journal of Marriage and the Family,* 1980, *42*(1), 9–15.

Shedd, C. W. *Grandparents: Then God created grandparents and it was very good.* Garden City, NY: Doubleday, 1976.

Sherman, S. R. Patterns of contacts for residents of age-segregated and age integrated housing. *Journal of Gerontology,* 1975, *30,* 103–107.

Sherman, S. R. Mutual assistance and support in retirement housing. *Journal of Gerontology*, 1975, *30*, 479–483.

Sherudi, E. *Grandma strikes back.* New York: Frederick Fell, 1979.

Soldo, B. J. America's elderly in the 1980's. *Population Bulletin*, 1980, *35*, 1–47.

Stephens, J. *Loners, losers, and lovers: Elderly tenants in a slum hotel.* Seattle: University of Washington Press, 1976.

Stinnett, N., Carter, L. M., and Montgomery, J. E. Older persons' perceptions of their marriages. *Journal of Marriage and the Family*, 1972, *34*, 665–670.

Streib, G. F., and Beck, R. W. Older families: A decade review. *Journal of Marriage and the Family*, 1980, *42*, 937–956.

Stueve, A., and Fischer, C. S. Social networks and older women. Working paper No. 292, University of California (Berkeley) Institute of Urban and Regional Development, 1978.

Stueve, C. A., and Lein, L. Problems in network analysis: The case of the missing elderly. Paper presented at the 32nd Annual Scientific Meeting of the Gerontological Society of America, Washington, DC, November 1979. Working Paper No. 50, Wellesley College Center for Research on Women.

Sussman, M. B., and Burchinal, L. Parental aid to married children: Implications for family functioning. Marriage and Family Living, 1962, *24*, 320–332.

Thompson, G. B. Aged women, OASDI beneficiaries: Income and characteristics, 1971. *Social Security Bulletin*, 1977, *40*, 23–48.

Tobin, S. S., and Kulys, R. The Family and services. In C. Eisdorfer et al. (Eds.), *Annual review of gerontology and geriatrics*, Vol. 1. New York: Springer, 1980.

Treas, J. Family support systems for the aged: Some social and demographic considerations. *The Gerotologist*, 1977, *17*, 486-491.

Troll, L. E., Miller, S. J., and Atchley, R. C. *Families in Later Life.* Belmont, CA: Wadsworth, 1979.

Turner, B. F. The self-concepts of older women. *Research in Aging*, 1979, *1*, 464–480.

Vincente, L., Wiley, J. A., and Carrington, R. A. The risk of institutionalization before death. *The Gerontologist*, 1974, *19*, 361–367.

Wan, T. T. H. Effects of family and informal networks on the use of skilled nursing facilities among the disabled elderly. Paper presented at the 33rd Annual Scientific Meeting of the Gerontological Society of America, San Diego, November 1980.

WCVB. What should be done about mom and dad? Channel 5, Boston, 1981.

Wentowski, G. J. Old age in an urban setting: Coping strategies, reciprocity, and personal networks. Paper presented at the 32nd Annual Scientific Meeting of the Gerontological Society of America, Washington, DC, November 1979.

Wilcox, B. L. Social support in adjusting to marital disruption: A network analysis. In B. H. Gottlieb (Ed.), *Social networks and social support.* Beverly Hills, CA: Sage, 1981.

Woehrer, C. E. Cultural pluralism in American families: The influence of ethnicity in social aspects of aging. *The Family Coordinator*, 1978, *27*, 329–339.

The Impact of Poverty
on Social Networks and Supports

Deborah E. Belle

Observers of city life have given us contradictory pictures of social relationships in poor neighborhoods. According to writers such as Sennett (1970), the material scarcities of urban ghettoes lead to sharing and to direct contact with others in the same situation. Such sharing and face-to-face interaction lead, in turn, to a "feeling of community, of being related and bound together in some way" (p. 48). The urban ghetto resident can thus experience a solidarity with peers, a warmth and a sense of community which people from more affluent neighborhoods can only envy. At the same time, the voluntary sharing of goods helps assure a sense of economic security. On the other hand, writers such as Rainwater (1970) and Liebow (1967) describe interpersonal relationships among the urban poor as "tentative," "ambivalent" and "shifting." They argue that the stresses of poverty endanger marriages and friendships and undercut the efforts of men and women to maintain these relationships.

Have the social ties of poor men and women been overly romanticized by some, or viewed too cynically by others? Is there something enviable in the communal experiences of the poor, or does material deprivation weaken social ties? Do poor families benefit from effective social support networks? After an introductory discussion of the relationships among stress, support and social relationships, this article explores the social networks of the urban poor and discusses the experiences of low-income women who rear children. Attention is focused on those who live at or slightly above the poverty level, rather than on stable working class families. As Liem and Liem (1978) have argued, "interpersonal relationships occur within broader social contexts" (p. 150).

Deborah E. Belle is Assistant Professor, Department of Psychology, Boston University.

For the poor, economic stress has a large role in shaping these contexts.

STRESS

While stress has been defined in diverse ways, most discussions of stress refer to a process in which an individual experiences threats to well-being which, at least temporarily, exhaust available resources, leading to negative outcomes. Most stress researchers therefore consider: (1) sources of stress, which are often called "stressors," (2) moderators of stress, including the resources used to master stressors, and (3) manifestations of stress, such as physical or mental ill health or family problems (Pearlin et al., 1982).

While there is a tradition of experimental, laboratory research on stress, most research on human reactions to naturally occurring stressors relies on questionnaire, interview, or archival data (either prospective or retrospective) to explore associations between presumed stressors, moderators and manifestations of stress. While these methodologies must leave one cautious about attributing causality to the correlational findings which emerge, the weight of corroboratory evidence which has accumulated over the past years of research does produce considerable confidence in several lines of inquiry. In addition, several intensive, participant observation studies complement the survey research which has been undertaken, and such intensive studies often point to the contexts and processes which lie behind the empirical relationships demonstrated in other studies.

SOCIAL SUPPORT

Social support, defined as emotional and instrumental assistance from others, has been perhaps the most widely researched moderator of stress. While social-support researchers have worked without a universally accepted definition of social support and without a standard social-support measure of proven reliability and validity, their work has generated massive evidence that the provision of emotional and instrumental assistance does buffer individuals in a wide variety of stressful situations (Cobb, 1976; Finlayson, 1976; Burke and Weir, 1977; Dean and Lin, 1977; Unger and Powell, 1980; McCubbin et al., 1980). Researchers have found, for instance, that social support is protective of the physical and mental health of men who lose their jobs (Gore, 1978) and protects women under stress from complications of pregnancy (Nuckolls et al., 1972). The quality of the mother-child relationship has also been found to reflect the social support available to the mother. Such support may come from the spouse (Hetherington et al., 1978), from other important figures such as the mother's own mother (Feiring and Taylor, n.d.), and from the network of kin and friends (Unger and Powell, 1980; Abernethy, 1973). Child abuse has been found to be most prevalent when parents are not only stressed, but also isolated (Garbarino, 1976).

THE COSTS OF SOCIAL TIES

While the positive impact of supportive social ties has thus been well documented, there is also evidence that not all social ties provide social support. Furthermore, there are often costs associated with maintaining membership in a social network composed of family members, friends, and others with whom regular contact is maintained.

In a study of psychiatric and medical patients, Tolsdorf (1976) found that many of the life stresses reported by respondents actually originated primarily in the social network, when "friends, family, or employers expected a certain role performance that the individual was unable to deliver. Failure to perform resulted in negative consequences and an increase in anxiety. As anxiety increased, performance dropped, inducing a vicious circle" (p. 414). When confronted with this type of stress, many respondents responded with "therapeutic withdrawal" and avoided further stress by reducing contact with network members. While this strategy can be viewed as adaptive, it also deprived respondents of potential support from network members.

Straus (1980) has reported that family violence is actually more prevalent among couples who have many relatives living nearby than among couples who are geographically isolated from their kin. Straus notes that this finding contradicts our usual assumption that "the network will be prosocial. That is usually a reasonable assumption. However, a social network can also support antisocial behavior" (p. 246). Several of Straus' respondents noted that when they left their husbands because of violent attacks, their own mothers urged them to adjust to the situation and to tolerate it for the sake of the children. In a similar vein, Collins and Pancoast (1976) note the existence of "negative networks" which promote destructive behavior such as alcohol dependence and delinquency. They point out that while such networks have destructive potential, they also serve important functions for their members which should not be ignored and should be replaced if individuals are to disengage themselves from such networks.

The mother-child relationship has been found to suffer when there are stressful social interactions between the mother and members of her social network, just as it appears to benefit from the positive social support to the mother. Hetherington et al. (1978) found that when divorced parents were in conflict and had disagreements about their children, frequent visits by the noncustodial father were associated with poor mother-child functioning and with disruptions in the child's behavior. Similarly, Wahler (1980) found that among isolated low-income mothers with problems in childrearing, days marked by visits from critical or controlling relatives were also days on which mothers were likely to have more negative interactions with their children.

Heavy involvement in a social network which is otherwise benign may still produce negative consequences. Cohler and Lieberman (1981) discovered that for middle-aged women in certain ethnic groups, having extensive social ties was associated with an overload of responsibility and with heightened psychological distress. The demands of network members appeared to be more draining than rewarding to these women. Eckenrode and Gore (1981) found that women whose network members experienced stressful life events such as illnesses or burglaries reported finding these events stressful, and even reflected this vicarious stress in their own poor health outcomes.

A specific type of network may entail both costs and benefits for individual participants. For instance, Abernethy (1973) found that a tightly knit network in which each member knew the other members and maintained frequent contact with them was associated with a confident approach to childrearing, while "women in loose networks appear to suffer from insufficient feedback, and are likely to be exposed to a confusing array of variants in childrearing theory" (p. 86). Yet Granovetter (1973) has shown that the individual who is enmeshed in a tightly knit network can be dangerously isolated from new ideas, information and mobility opportunities.

A network in which members rely heavily on each other for emotional or material support may provide crucial resources in times of need and yet may also strain itself to the breaking point. As Tietjen (1980) has noted, "Some individuals may have excessive demands made on them by their network members, or families with limited material or emotional resources may become overly indebted to their network members, a condition that they may find uncomfortable. These and other situations can strain a mutually supportive relationship to the point of dissolution" (pp. 18-19).

Thus, a social network does not automatically constitute a social support network to its members. Some members of the network may constitute a net drain on emotional and material resources, and other social ties may be both supportive and stressful at the same time. A network which provides consensus and community may not provide fresh ideas or new opportunities. Social relationships can be both stressful and supportive.

POVERTY

Poverty is one of the most potent stressors known to social science. Low income means high risk for mental health problems (Warheit et al., 1976; Brown et al., 1975; Liem and Liem, 1978; Dohrenwend and Dohrenwend, 1965; Srole et al., 1962), poor physical health (Children's Defense Fund, 1979) and family violence (Pelton, 1978; Garbarino, 1976; Garbarino and Sherman, 1980; Straus, 1980). After reviewing 22 studies in which stress was a dependent variable, Weisner and Abbott (1977) conclude that there is "a near universal tendency for low socioeconomic status or low income to be associated with high stress" (p. 445). Only in socialist Sweden was an exception found to this general principle. The authors note, "The Swedes seem to have managed a reversal in one of the most consistently patterned relationships reported in the literature" (p. 445). While many studies claim that poverty is a stressor through the kind of correlational analysis discussed earlier, time-series analyses such as those of Brenner (1973) lend considerable credibility to the argument.

Not only does poverty impose considerable stress on individuals, it also attacks many potential sources of social support and sets some of the conditions under which social support can be provided to buffer individuals against stress. In particular, poverty appears to threaten marriages. It exposes individuals to a high level of "contagion of stress" when their network members suffer poverty-related life events and stressful life conditions. Poor men and women often must deal with "negative networks" in their own neighborhoods. Poverty also forces many individuals to engage in survival networks which preclude upward mobility and which often exact emotional penalties. "Therapeutic withdrawal" from network ties is often an adaptive, though costly, response to the stress of social networks among the poor.

Marital solidarity appears to be more difficult to maintain among the poor than among the more affluent. Parents living below the poverty line are less likely to be happily married than those above the poverty line (Zill, 1978), and women in families of lower socioeconomic status are less likely to turn to their husbands as confidants (Brown et al., 1975). Men who provide very low or sporadic income for their families are likely candidates for marital dissolution and divorce (Cherlin, 1979), and among families living at or below the poverty level, husband-wife families are drastically underrepresented. Half of all families living in poverty do not include a husband-father (U.S. Bureau of the Census, 1980).

Poverty also severely limits the extent to which individuals can exercise choice in matters relevant to potential stress and social support. Compared to more affluent city dwellers, poor men and women exercise little choice about where and among whom to live. Buying power and renting power are limited by poverty, of course. Those who must depend on public housing or on publicly subsidized housing are further limited in their choice of a residential location. Discrimination against racial and ethnic minorities, single parent families and families with many children often sets up additional barriers, so that the decision about where to locate is hardly a choice at all.

Not surprisingly, the urban poor are generally not strongly enamored of their own neighborhoods or neighbors. A study of poor women in Harlem found that women were more likely to rate the block where they lived a poor place to live than a fair or good place, and that their children were even more likely than they to view the immediate neighborhood negatively (Gordon, 1965). Only a third of the children who were interviewed named any positive attribute of their block when asked specifically what they liked about it. Rainwater (1970) found that most residents of a federal housing project held "dim views of the project community" (p. 101). More recently, Belle (1982) found that when urban low-income mothers rated their neighborhoods on attributes like personal safety, quietness, protection of property, and sense of community, they rarely chose the highest rating (very good), and on average rated community characteristics somewhere between "not so good" and "good." Furthermore, women who had lived in the same neighborhood for longer periods of time were no more likely than relative newcomers to rate the neighborhood positively, suggesting that the lack of enthusiasm for the neighborhood was not an effect of transience and that women who remained displeased with their neighborhoods found themselves unable to move to preferred locations.

The poor also generally have less ability than those with more wealth to defend the boundaries of their own neighborhoods against outside interference. Urban renewal efforts are often launched against neighborhoods which do not appear to the residents of these neighborhoods to be slums in need of clearance. The poor generally lack the powerful political contacts which could prevent the displacement of their communities and the destruction of the buildings in which they still wish to live. Those with more wealth can also simply buy out the poor or raise property values and taxes until the poor are forced to leave. Nor do the poor generally have the economic or political power to keep "undesirables" out of their neighborhoods. Crime is a frequent concomitant of poverty, and many low-income areas are also high-crime areas. This means high levels of personal victimization for individuals and high levels of "stress contagion" when members of the social network experience such victimization.

A recent study of victimization in a small urban housing project found that almost half of the surveyed households had experienced a robbery, burglary or assault against one of their members (Merry, 1981). Belle et al. (1981) reported that a sample of 42 urban low-income mothers had experienced a total of 37 violent events (crime, sexual assault, household violence) during the two-year period preceding the study, and these same respondents reported an additional 35 violent events which had happened to network members who were important to them.

"Negative networks" in the immediate neighborhood can be highly stressful to poor families, particulary to those with children. In their studies of urban housing projects, both Merry (1981) and

Rainwater (1970) found many parents fearful that their children would be tempted away from respectability by the glamorous and exciting "street life" going on around them. While parents often tried to isolate their children from those involved with crime, hustling and drugs, the enterprise often proved futile. What incentives could parents offer children which could compete with the easy money and excitement of the illicit activities they saw going on around them? The efforts of parents to protect their children from dangerous influences often isolated families in their own apartments and divided neighbors from each other. Yet, even if young children could be effectively cloistered and chaperoned, attempts at such control generally crumbled during adolescence.

While isolation and retreat from "the street" represent one strategy of response to urban poverty, the development of an informal network of mutual aid is also a frequent adaptation to poverty. (These strategies may even involve the same individuals. A person may seek isolation from neighbors while relying on a network of kinfolk and friends for mutual assistance.) Stack's classic participant observation study (1974) describes such mutual aid networks among low-income black women. For the women Stack studied, their meager incomes from welfare and from poorly paid work barely covered the necessities of life: food, clothing and shelter. No surplus cash remained to meet unexpected losses and crises, such as illnesses, robberies, or late welfare checks. Therefore, informal exchange networks were created among kin and trusted friends to provide mutual aid when the inevitable crises arose. Without such help, no individual or family could long survive. The women Stack studied gave each other goods, money and assistance when they could, and, in turn, they received help when they were themselves in need. In this way, no one faced a serious crisis alone, and each participant in the mutual aid network had a virtual insurance policy to buffer the stress of such crises.

While these mutual aid networks ensured survival in a hostile environment, they also exacted costs. Some individuals appeared to take advantage of the generosity of others and failed to respond with the expected reciprocal generosity. Other network members suffered when they found themselves so deeply indebted to others that they could not legitimately resist unwelcome intrusions into their lives by those to whom they were indebted. One woman, for instance, had relied extensively on a kinswoman for child care assistance and realized that she would have to rely on this woman's help in the future as well. She found herself powerless to prevent this kinswoman from disciplining and even terrifying her children in her own presence in ways she disliked. To protest or even to withdraw from this kinswoman would have left the mother and her children dangerously unprepared for future crises.

While Stack regards the networks she observed and participated in as a remarkable survival strategy, she also notes that such networks effectively preclude upward mobility and an escape from poverty. "Few if any black families living on welfare for the second generation are able to accumulate a surplus of the basic necessities to be able to remove themselves from poverty or from the collective demands of kin" (p. 33, underlining added). Any cash surpluses which network members acquire are quickly distributed throughout the network, reducing the original possessors to the common poverty level from which they started. In order to remove themselves from poverty, individuals must break with the mutual aid network that assured their survival in poverty.

There is evidence that among the urban poor it is those who are most hardpressed who enter most completely into such networks of mutual aid. Stack found that those women in a position to do without the exchanges of the network because of secure access to economic resources tended to opt out of the mutual obligations that such exchanges entailed. Similarly, Jeffers (1967) reported that in the public housing project where she conducted her own participant observations, the most extensive involvements with neighbors were maintained by those families with especially "inadequate and uncertain incomes" and those for whom "the task of keeping a roof over their heads and food in their children's mouths occupied much of their time" (p. 19). Recently, Belle (1982) found that, among low-income urban mothers, those experiencing more stressful life circumstances involved themselves more frequently in exchange and socializing with their neighbors. Such findings suggest that while mutual aid networks are critical as a survival strategy among the poor, they are not voluntarily chosen by those who can find other means to assure survival and even escape from poverty.

SOCIAL SUPPORT AND LOW-INCOME MOTHERS

In recent years, we have become increasingly aware of the stresses involved in rearing young children on a low income. Several studies have found, for instance, that low-income mothers are at great risk for depression (Brown et al., 1975; Pearlin and John-son, 1977; Radloff, 1975). The forms of socal support which can protect low-income mothers from mental health problems such as depression are thus of special interest.

Several studies have found that low-income mothers who have at least one close and confiding relationship are buffered against the stresses of their situation. Belle (1982) found that low-income mothers who were able to discuss their feelings with someone were less likely to experience depression than women without such confidants. Brown et al. (1975) reported, however, that only con-fiding relationships with spouses or boyfriends were protective for women.

The importance of emotional support for the mother-child rela-tionship has also been demonstrated. Feiring and Taylor (n.d.) found that a mother's involvement and responsivity with her infant were positively associated with emotional support from the spouse or from another important figure such as the mother's own mother. The authors present their results within the context of attachment theory, noting that the types of maternal behavior which are asso-ciated with strong support are also those which foster secure at-tachment between mother and child. Longfellow et al. (1979) found, however, that the extent of emotional support available to low-income mothers of young children was not associated with maternal behavior patterns observed in the home. The discrepancy between these two studies may relate to the age of the child in each: Feiring and Taylor studied mothers of infants, while Longfellow et al. studied mothers of older children. It is also pos-sible that the different findings are attributable to the different ways in which the researchers measured emotional support.

Belle (1982) found that not only emotional support, but also daily help with routine tasks and assistance with child care were positively related to mental health among low-income mothers with young children. Such support often came from friends and relatives as well as from husbands and boyfriends. Of all the types of social support studied, routine child care was related to the most indicators of mental health, suggesting that this may be a particu-larly important form of social support for women rearing young children with low incomes. Longfellow et al. (1979) also found that assistance with child care, particularly when this assistance came from other adults, was associated with positive aspects of observed maternal behavior. The extent of help with daily tasks did not, however, predict observed maternal behavior. An unpublished study by Unger, reported by Unger and Powell (1980) discovered that mothers who received material resources from others were also more responsive to their children.

SOCIAL NETWORKS AND SOCIAL SUPPORT AMONG LOW-INCOME MOTHERS

While the importance of social support to low-income mothers has thus been documented, and some of the specific types of crucial social support have been located, questions remain about the types of social networks which most adequately provide social support to low-income mothers. Is a large social network the key to effective social support? Or do the costs of social ties detract from the social support which such ties offer?

The unpublished study by Unger reported by Unger and Powell (1980) found that frequent contact with kin and friends was characteristic of mothers who were actively involved with their infants. Such a finding suggests that the social network is socially supportive. Yet Belle (1982) found no evidence that low-income mothers who lived near to and interacted frequently with many relatives and friends experienced mental health advantages over more isolated women. While the socially involved women received more emotional and instrumental support than did the isolated women, they also reported significantly more stress about their relatives and friends than did the women with smaller social networks. Women reported problems with physical and verbal abuse, betrayed confidences, and overwhelming demands for assistance. Many of the women in the study appeared to be providing far more instrumental and emotional support to others than they received in return. Even when relationships were not problematic in these ways, the women often worried about their relatives' and friends' problems with poor health, difficult relationships, or troubling housing situations. The social networks of the women Belle studied appeared to provide stress and support in almost equal quantities, so that there was no net advantage to a larger social network. It is difficult to reconcile the Unger findings with those of Belle. Assuming that the discrepant findings represent genuine differences in the social networks studied by Unger and Belle and not methodological artifacts, it would be important to investigate further the factors which enable the social networks of some low-income mothers to provide more support than stress, while the networks of other women in similar circumstances appear to be as draining as they are supportive.

While Belle and Unger took global measures of each respondent's social network involvement, Wahler (1980) obtained measures of social network contact on specific days and compared these measurements with an assessment of maternal behavior observed on the same days. In addition to this important methodological innovation, Wahler obtained reports from the women he studied on the valence of social interactions (aversive to positive) so that he could distinguish those social contacts mothers enjoyed from those they found unpleasant. Wahler's target population was a sample of isolated low-income mothers who were experiencing problems in childrearing. His data revealed that day-to-day fluctuations in maternal behavior reflected day-to-day fluctuations in the social contacts mothers experienced. On days marked by enjoyable visits from friends, mothers were noticeably more positive to their children. Not only were mothers more positive on such days, but children also were more positive to their mothers. When mothers only experienced contacts with relatives they found critical and controlling, their maternal behavior suffered. Thus, the quality of the social contact was more important than the quantity of contacts mothers experienced.

CONCLUSIONS

Stress not only threatens individuals directly, it also can attack potential sources of social support which might otherwise be used to buffer that stress. The stresses of poverty appear to constrain social networks in many ways, making it difficult to draw from them the resources necessary to good mental health and family functioning. Research suggests that marital solidarity often suffers under the stresses of poverty, that neighborhoods often fail to provide a supportive context in which to live and rear children, and that social ties often provide poor people with vicarious stress and burdensome dependence while limiting mobility opportunities. There appear to be poignant conflicts between the pressing survival needs of the poor and their other needs for independence and autonomy.

Such findings suggest that future research should pay more attention to the costs as well as to the benefits of social networks.

The isolated woman may be one who has chosen "therapeutic withdrawal" from a demanding and draining network. For her, it may not be desirable to increase network contacts, at least not with the individuals who originally formed her network. More attention should be paid to the decisions individuals make about their networks and the rationales for these decisions. Both retreat and heavy involvement may be adaptive strategies for minimizing stress and maximizing support while living in poverty.

Since the natural helping networks of the poor are often emotionally costly, they should not be viewed as a substitute for formal helping networks or for economic security. The woman who must rely on a relative to care for her children may experience considerable emotional stress, while the woman who can find an affordable day care center or babysitter can suddenly moderate some of the stress in her life. This argument does not imply that paid babysitters are inherently more desirable than unpaid help. In fact, most women probably prefer a known and trusted relative or friend to a less well-known person they must pay. The argument is only intended to call to attention the plight of the woman whose economically enforced interdependence with network members is highly stressful and inescapable.

While this article has drawn attention to the ways in which poverty contrains and disrupts social support, it is also true that in other ways poverty may facilitate social support. Members of the middle class, for instance, may find fewer natural opportunities for sharing, since their own households are more self-sufficient than are those of the poor. It may also be that the desire to uphold a prestigious social position militates against help-seeking in times of trouble among the middle class. These propositions could be systematically tested.

In casting a cold eye on the social networks of poor men and women, this article has attempted to articulate the distinction between a social network and a social support network. While social support is a powerful buffer against stress, many social networks are no buffer at all, and actually contribute to the stress their participants experience.

REFERENCES

Abernethy, V. Social network and response to the maternal role. *International Journal of Sociology of the Family*, 1973, *3*, 86-92.

Belle, D. Social ties and social support. In D. Belle (Ed.), *Lives in stress: Women and depression.* Beverly Hills, California: Sage, 1982.

Belle, D. with C. Longfellow, V. Makosky, E. Saunders, and P. Zelkowitz. Income, mothers' mental health, and family functioning in a low-income population. In American Academy of Nursing, *The impact of changing resources on health policy.* Kansas City: American Academy of Nursing, 1981.

Brenner, M. H. *Mental illness and the economy.* Cambridge: Harvard University Press, 1973.

Brown, G., Bhrolchain, M. and Harris, T. Social class and psychiatric disturbance among women in an urban population. *Sociology,* 1975, *9*(2), 225-254.

Burke, R. and Weir, T. Marital helping relationships: The moderators between stress and well-being. *The Journal of Psychology,* 1977, *95,* 121-130.

Cherlin, A. Work life and marital dissolution. In G. Levinger and O. Moles (Eds.), *Divorce and separation: Context, causes and consequences.* New York: Basic Books, 1979.

Children's Defense Fund. America's children and their families, 1979.

Cobb, S. Social support as a moderator of life stress. *Psychosomatic Medicine,* 1976, *38*(5), 300-314.

Cohler, B. and Lieberman, M. Social relations and mental health among three European ethnic groups. *Research on Aging,* 1981, forthcoming.

Collins, A. and Pancoast, D. *Natural helping networks.* Washington, D.C.: National Association of Social Workers, 1976.

Dean, A. and Lin, N. The stress-buffering role of social support. *The Journal of Nervous and Mental Disease,* 1977, *165*(6), 403-417.

Dohrenwend, B. P. and Dohrenwend, B. S. The problem of validity in field studies of psychological disorder. *J. of Abnormal Psychology,* 1965, *70,* 52-69.

Eckenrode, J. and Gore, S. Stressful events and social support: The significance of context. In B. H. Gottlieb (Ed.), *Social netowrks and social support.* Beverly Hills: Sage, 1981.

Feiring, C. and Taylor, J. The influence of the infant and secondary parent on maternal behavior: Toward a social systems view of infant attachment. Unpublished paper. University of Pittsburgh.

Finlayson, A. Social networks as coping resources: Lay help and consultation patterns used by women in husbands' post-infarction career. *Soc. Sci. and Med.,* 1976, *10,* 97-103.

Garbarino, J. A preliminary study of some ecological correlates of child abuse: The impact of socioeconomic stress on mothers. *Child Dev.,* 1976, *47,* 178-185.

Garbarino, J. and Sherman, D. Identifying high-risk neighborhoods. In J. Garbarino, S. H. Stocking, and associates, *Protecting children from abuse and neglect: Developing and maintaining effective support systems for families.* San Francisco: Jossey-Bass, 1980.

Gordon, J. The poor of Harlem: Social functioning in the underclass. New York: Welfare Admin. Project 105, 1965.

Gore, S. The effect of social support in moderating the health consequences of unemployment. *J. of Health and Social Behavior,* 1978, *19,* 157-165.

Granovetter, M. The strength of weak ties. *Am. J. of Sociology,* 1973, *78*(6), 1360-1380.

Hetherington, E., Cox, M. and Cox, R. The aftermath of divorce. In J. H. Stevens, Jr. and M. Mathews (Eds.), *Mother-child father-child relationships.* Washington, D.C.: National Association for the Education of Young Children, 1978.

Liebow, E. *Tally's corner: A study of Negro streetcorner men.* Boston: Little, Brown and Co., 1967.

Liem, R. and Liem, J. Social class and mental illness reconsidered: The role of economic stress and social support. *J. of Health and Social Behavior,* 1978, *19,* 139-156.

Longfellow, C., Zelkowitz, P., Saunders, E., and Belle, D. The role of support in moderating the effects of stress and depression. Paper presented at the Biennial Meeting of the Society for Research in Child Development, San Francisco, March 15-18, 1979.

McCubbin, H., Joy, C., Cauble, A., Comeau, J., Patterson, J. and Needle, R. Family stress and coping: A decade review. *Journal of Marriage and the Family,* 1980, *42*(4), 855-871.

Merry, S. *Urban danger: Life in a neighborhood of strangers.* Philadelphia: Temple University Press, 1981.

Nuckolls, K., Cassel, J. and Kaplan, B. Psychosocial assets, life crisis and the prognosis of pregnancy. *Amer. J. Epidemiol.,* 1972, *95,* 431-441.

Pearlin, L. and Johnson, J. Marital status, life-strains and depression. *Am. Soc. Review,* 1977, *42,* 704-715.

Pearlin, L., Lieberman, M., Menaghan, E., and Mullan, J. The stress process. *J. of Health and Social Behavior,* 1982, forthcoming.

Pelton, L. Child abuse and neglect: The myth of classlessness, *Amer. J. Orthopsychiatry,* 1978, *48*(4), 608-617.

Radloff, L. Sex differences in depression: The effects of occupation and marital status. *Sex Roles: A Journal of Research,* 1975, *1,* 249-266.

Rainwater, L. *Behind ghetto walls: Black family life in a federal slum.* Chicago: Aldine, 1970.

Sennett, R. *The uses of disorder: Personal identity and city life.* New York: Vintage Books, 1970.

Srole, L., Langner, T., Michael, S., Opler, M., and Rennie, T. *Mental health in the metropolis: The Midtown Manhattan Study, Vol. I.* New York: McGraw-Hill, 1962.

Straus, M. Social stress and marital violence in a national sample of American families. *Annals of the New York Academy of Sciences,* 1980, *347,* 229-250.

Tietjen, A. Integrating formal and informal support systems: The Swedish experience. In J. Garbarino, S. H. Stocking, and associates, *Protecting children from abuse and neglect: Developing and maintaining effective support systems for families.* San Francisco: Jossey-Bass, 1980.

Tolsdorf, C. Social networks, support, and coping: An exploratory study. *Family Process,* 1976, *15*(2), 407-417.

Unger, D. and Powell, D. Supporting families under stress: The role of social networks. *Family Relations,* 1980, *29,* 566-574.

U.S. Bureau of the Census, Current Population Reports, Series P-60, No. 125. *Money income and poverty status of families and persons in the United States: 1979 (Advance Report).* U.S. Government Printing Office, Washington, D.C., 1980.

Wahler, R. The insular mother: Her problems in parent-child treatment. *J. of Applied Behavior Analysis,* 1980, *13,* 207-219.

Warheit, G., Holzer, C., Bell, R. and Arey, S. Sex, marital status, and mental health: A reappraisal. *Social Forces,* 1976, *55,* 2, 459-470.

Weisner, T. and Abbott, S. Women, modernity and stress: Three contrasting contexts for change in East Africa. *J. of Anthropological Research,* 1977, *33*(4), 421-451.

Zill, N. Divorce, marital happiness and the mental health of children. Findings from the CCD National Survey of Children. Unpublished report, 1978.

NOTE

This article was written with the support of grant number MH28830 of the Mental Health Services Development Branch of the National Institute of Mental Health, Susan Salasin, Project Officer.

Analytic Essay:
The Ties that Bind

Kris Jeter

Family ties have various strengths, weaknesses, meanings, and knots. In this analytic essay I discuss five recently published books that define these ties, present the emotional costs and benefits, and describe therapy which uses these ties. The unique psychologies of father and son; grandmother, mother, and daughter; and sibling ties are investigated. A journal written by a daughter as primary caretaker for two parents fighting life threatening disease illustrates the emotions of crisis networking. Lastly a therapeutic application of social network intervention is abstracted.

In 1982, Lee Salk, child psychologist, wrote *My Father, My Son: Intimate Relationships.* In-depth interviews consisting of freeform and open-ended questions were conducted with men representing varied careers, ethnicity, geographic locations, and socioeconomic classes. Salk presents, in Studs Terkel style, 28 psychological portraits of father-son relationships; some span four generations.

Salk reputes Freud's theory of the Oedipus complex which purports that the father-son relationship is constructed around anger, conflict, destructive impulses, hostility, jealousy, and resentment. Salk finds that fathers and sons either have or want affection, discipline, love, physical contact, tenderness, and time together. The son's sense of identity emerges from the father's recognition of his son's unique individuality. The most masculine boys view their fathers to be powerful and nurturing. Salk suggests that machismo is a man's reaction to an emotion about masculinity rather than a reflection of masculinity.

Recent research has addressed the question of father-infant relationships. Salk supports this trend and predicts accepted societal practices of four-day work weeks, househusbandry, paternity

Kris Jeter, PhD, is a Trainer, Human Development Specialist and Associate with Beacon Research Associates, Ltd., Inc.

leave, and shorter work days to free fathers, as well as mothers, for their parenting roles.

To me, these life stories also tell of the continuity of life over generations, the give and take in stressful as well as easy times. The constant bonding promotes stability and the active growth adds excitement. Father and sons are to feel love and support from each other throughout their life spans.

In 1981, psychologists Bertram J. Cohler and Henry U. Grunebaum explored the female parenting tie. In *Mothers, Grandmothers, and Daughters,* they indicate that even though there has been research which measures the amount of contact and support of kin across generations, the psychological significance of such support has been neglected in the literature.

The purpose of the research was to acquire quantitative data measuring personality and childcare attitudes of mothers and grandmothers residing together or living apart. These data could be used for comparison research and to determine a baseline for other studies on mothers and grandmothers. Cohler and Grunebaum administered the "Maternal Attitude Scale" and a "Family Information Form" to a sample of 90 grandmothers and their daughters who were mothers of at least one child below five years of age.

A clinical study was designed to provide insight on possible interpretation of these quantitative data. Four Catholic, Italian descent, urban-reared mother-grandmother pairs were selected to represent four categories of relationships: (1) appropriate closeness with more adaptive attitudes and living apart; (2) inappropriate closeness and less adaptive attitudes living apart; (3) appropriate closeness and more adaptive attitudes sharing a residence; and (4) inappropriate closeness and less adaptive attitudes and sharing a residence. The eight women responded to the "Thematic Apperception Test" and the "Interpersonal Apperception Technique" series. They also completed the "Minnesota Multiphasic Personality Inventory." Entire families were interviewed over a several-day period at the initiation of this clinical study and four years later.

There were three discrete results. (1) Daughters are socialized to maintain interpendent relationships with their mother. In adulthood similar interests and sentiments deepen the interdependency. (2) Different developmental stages may be the cause for the feeling of discomfort grandmothers experience when asked by daughters to babysit and assist. Mothers experience overload in their roles as caretaker for dependent offspring, daughter, homemaker, kin-keeper, and wife. New mothers will seek assistance and support from their own mothers while developing an independence from her. Meanwhile their mother is concerned with the developmental task of interiority and strive to deepen her inner harmony and integrity. The mother-toddler age daughter relationship is quite different from the mother-childbearing age daughter relationships. (3) Multigeneration adult families do relate across generations socially and psychologically. This interdependence is a significant fountainhead for personal congruence, ego strength, and identity. Cross generational interdependence causes conflict only when personalities merge. The quality of the grandmother's continuing socialization is more significant to the multigenerational family than residence. Conflict was most evident in the one multigenerational family in which the two generations lived a great distance apart. The extent to which adults adapt to life events which require human care and love best determines relatedness. Interdependency and loyalty rather than individuality should be the task of the therapist.

Four years later, changes between mothers and grandmothers appeared to result from external circumstances rather than personality developmental changes. The young mothers desired intimate relationships with their mothers. Their mothers, now grandmothers, experienced discomfort about the close psychological ties. Granddaughters of hostile, close intergenerational families adjust with more difficulty than granddaughters of interdependent, tolerant intergenerational families.

Cohler and Grunebaum's concept of adaptation to life events facilitating interdependence and loyalty is illustrated in *Caring: A Daughter's Story*. In 1978, at the age of 42, Diane Rubin, a professional writer, became the primary caretaker for her mother with cancer and her father, a stroke victim. She highlights portions of a journal she kept into her 1982 book for lay and professional readers. With approval of her family, Rubin shares her emotions during this three-year period of her life of being on 24-hour call. Anger, bewilderment, exhaustion, fear, impatience, jealousy, tension, and terror are balanced with affection, care, concern, duty, gratitude, kindness, love, and patience. At first, Rubin would cry many times throughout the day wherever she was without embarrassment or apology. A year later the tears stopped and a numbness set in. Rubin fights for control of the setting, feeling unable to control the diseases.

The dynamic interplay between members of her family network

is accented by the support of her sister, husband, and two teenage sons. During the first year, the family enters into five weeks of group therapy. Secrets are told; battles are fought; affection, pride, and strength are disclosed and recognized.

Rubin yearns for a normal life-style, for sleep. She meets a friend who is also a primary caretaker of her parents. They share their complaints and experiences with full knowledge that this conversation could be repeated by their own children twenty years hence.

Rubin reflects that suffering begets family strength—even when it is thought that the last bit has been expended. For herself, Rubin has revalued her life-style. Uncomplicated, honest, affectionate relationships matter. Diane Rubin is still Diane Rubin, however, more self-forgiving. She has learned that she has been "a good daughter" and "can be counted on."

Rubin unfolds the developmental stages of being a primary caretaker for adults facing life threatening disease in a factual and intimate way. Her book would be an asset to teachers of adult growth and development and caretaking families and teachers of any subject matter who encourage journal writing. Rubin devotes limited book space to her sister and their relationship.

In *The Sibling Bond,* a 1982 publication by clinical psychologists Stephen P. Bank and Michael D. Kahn do attend to the relationships between brothers and sisters. Clinical training ignores the influence of siblings on each other. Parents are thought to form a child's identity and from there on the job, spouse, and children provide the chart for an adult's life course.

The authors reviewed five areas of literature and provided brief descriptions of their findings. Psychoanalysts wrote of sibling rivalry. Twin researchers entangled twin's emotions with each other. Family systems theorists classified children into one subgroup and parents into another subgroup. Birth-order theorists have indicated that a person's order in birth dicates certain personality traits. Sociologists have examined commonalities of the sibling relationships. A holistic viewpoint or theory consensus was not found in the literature. Furthermore, few studies have concentrated concurrently on sibling and parent relationships; have investigated siblings in crisis circumstances; or have longitudinally examined siblings.

Historically, siblings who immigrated to the United States felt it necessary to maintain close contact with each other in order to retain their cultural heritage and to survive in an unfamiliar environment. Today, siblings are less likely to need each other for emotional and physical survival and will choose to be involved with each other. Emotions siblings may feel for each other may range from ambivalence to expressed love. Loss and adversity tend to create allies of siblings.

In the last century, changes in cultural patterns have stimulated the importance of sibling relationships. Small-size families concentrate the relationships of siblings to a lesser number and greater intensity. Two career parents may leave their children unsupervised together to entertain and care for each other. Children may be aware of their parents competing in the work world and adopt a competitive relationship with their sibling(s). Parents may experience severe stress, and siblings may turn to each other for sustenance. As adults, persons moving to new environments or engaged in divorce or remarriage may find that their sibling relationship provides a firm anchor in the turbulence. Extended lifetimes combined with a smaller number of siblings in a family may produce lonely aged people who, when the only survivor, may feel unlinked with either the past or present.

The sibling bond ties individuals together on both the intimate and the public levels. Even if there might be a personality clash, there still is a feeling of comfort established by a familiar, predictable presence, especially during life changes and crises.

Bank and Kahn explore siblings in different life stages, emotional and sexual states, and conflicts. They discuss sibling-specific therapeutic techniques. A clint may explore her or his family inheritance, alter the sibling bond, work through resentments, and understand personal developmental changes in light of sibling experiences. The therapist may isolate the client and invite, rally, or rehearse other siblings.

Counseling not only siblings but the entire family system is discussed in *Networking Family in Crisis* published in 1979. Uri Rueveni, family therapist and counseling psychologist, outlines for professional clinicians the social network intervention method called networking. Hunting and gathering societies needed networking for survival. Industrial societies have less effective extended families and therapeutic interventions have been substituted for the family. Networking conveys the flow, interactions, interdependence, linkage, and meshing of the group of people—family and non-family—who are most important to a client's life.

Family network intervention is goal-directed and time-limited. The objective is to assist family members to mobilize the social network support system in order to collectively develop new options for solving a crisis. This intervention process confirms the network phases Speck and Attneave have contributed to the literature: retribalization, polarization, mobilization, depression, breakthrough, and exhaustion-elation. During retribalization, people reconnect with known relatives and greet new family members. During polarization the family share their feelings and viewpoints about the crisis. Therapists are not to provide answers, but rather to encourage participation. Mobilization occurs when family activists lead small groups to investigate problem solving. During the depression stage, boredom, frustration, and tension can occur if acceptance of all members' contributions is not felt. At the time of breakthrough, positive action and feelings of optimism and encouragement propel the family toward actual problem-solving consensus. In exhaustion-elation, the last phase, the family is satisfied with their work together.

In this era, stereotyped as the new federalism, with institutional resources to provide human resources dwindling, there has been a rediscovery of the supportive networks. Rediscovered is an ongoing phenomenon which has existed during the period of recorded history. Supportive networks have been built around families and kin from time immemorial and where non-family and non-kin are involved and they are apt to be treated "like family." The writers of the books reviewed have implicitly or explicitly demonstrated that family and kin support networks are the ones individuals count on when in trouble or in need of affection, assistance, caring, instruction, love, and warmth. The consequences may not be optional in providing a quality life-style for the respondents and, in fact, the outcomes may be devastating economically and psychologically. Yet the network is there, it responds and can be responsive if nurtured and guided. This is what family and kin is all about!

BOOKS REVIEWED

Bank, Stephen P. and Michael D. Kahn. *The Sibling Bond.* New York: Basic Books, Inc., 1982.
Cohler, Bertram J. and Henry U. Grunebaum. *Mothers, Grandmothers, and Daughters:*

Personality and Childcare in Three-Generation Families. New York: John Wiley and Sons, 1981.

Rubin, Diane. *Caring: A Daughter's Story*. New York: Holt, Rinehart and Winston, 1982.

Rueveni, Uri. *Networking Families in Crisis: Intervention Strategies with Families and Social Networks*. New York: Human Sciences Press, 1979.

Salk, Lee. *My Father, My Son: Intimate Relationships*. New York: G. P. Putnam's Sons, 1982.

Speck, Ross V. and Attneave, C. *Family Networks*. New York: Vintage Books, 1973.